MW00583135

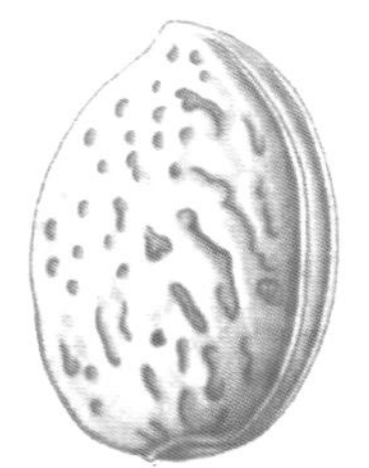

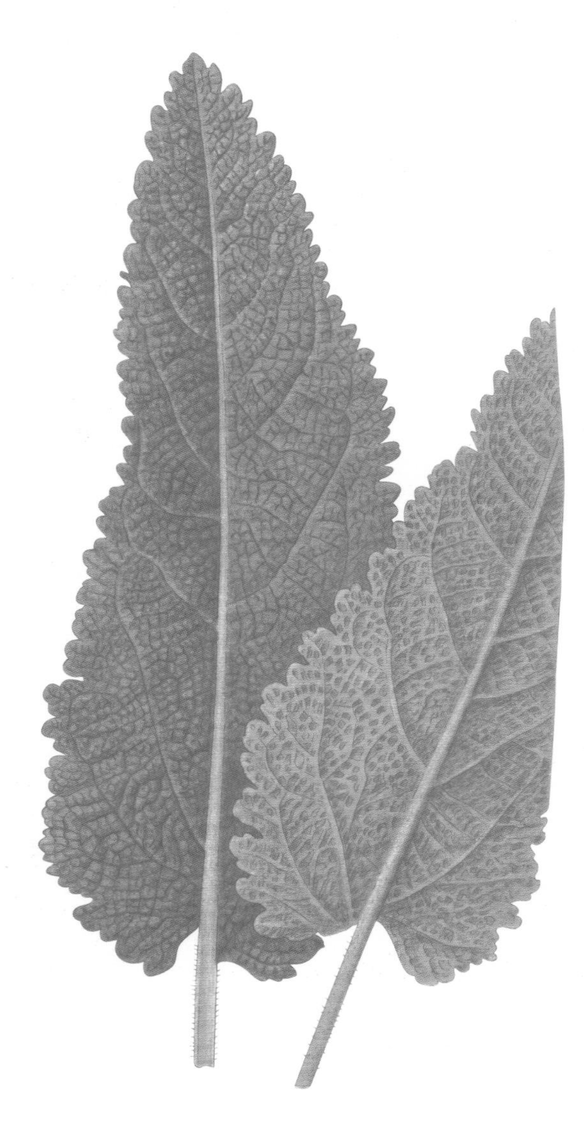

ANTI-INFLAMMATORY DIET SOLUTION

HEAL YOUR IMMUNE SYSTEM, BOOST YOUR BRAIN, STRENGTHEN YOUR HEART

Here's my collected advice for a healthier life—the complete story about the anti-inflammatory diet, good intestinal flora, and how to change your lifestyle

Stig Bengmark

English translation by Gun Penhoat

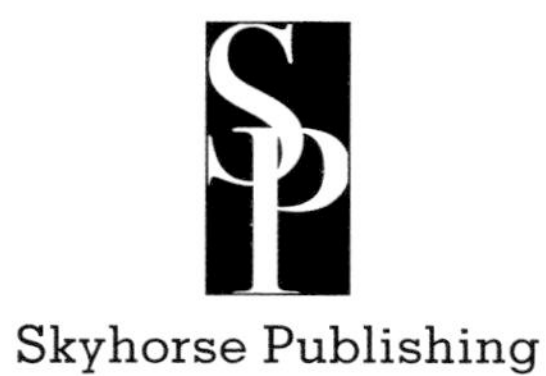

Skyhorse Publishing

03

Lifestyle and Diet Are Up to You 50

04

Three Basic Pillars: Exercise, Proper Diet, Stress Reduction 80

Foreword

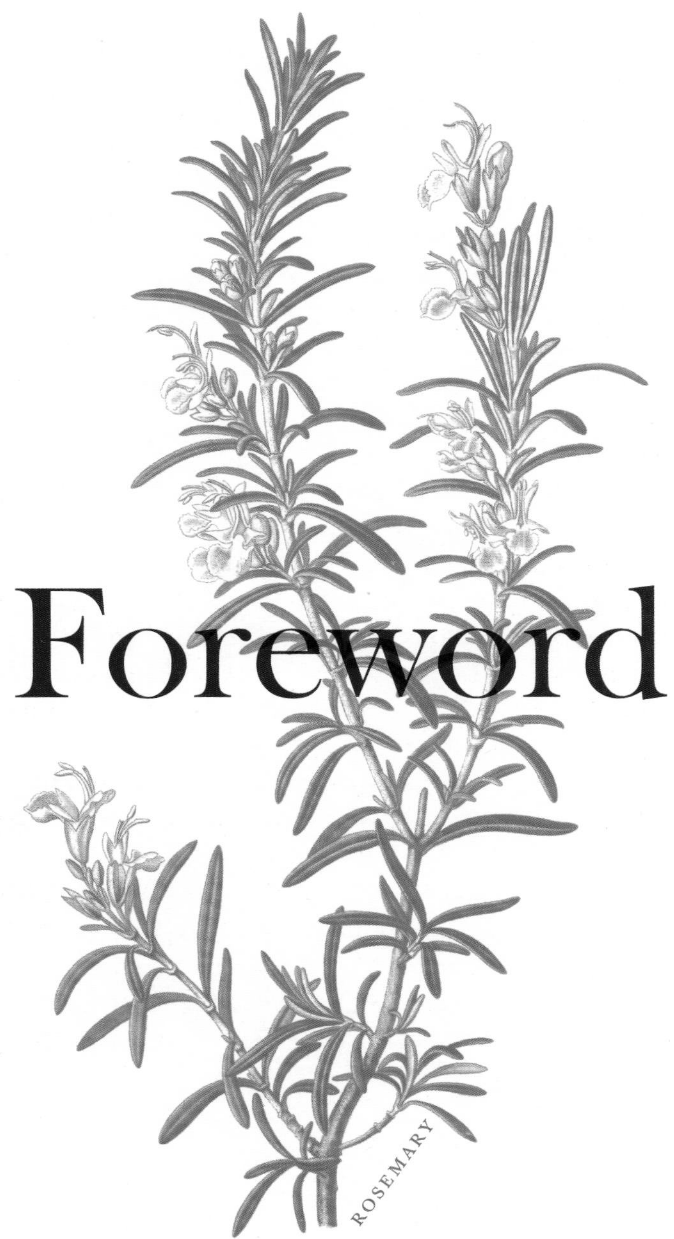

THE PICTURE OF a long-ago breakfast meeting pops up in my memory when Stig's name is mentioned. We are meeting in a hotel in Stockholm to plan research projects, and it is 8 o'clock on a Saturday morning.

Stig chose the hour for the meeting. I wondered quietly what would make the (then) eighty-five-year-old professor want to meet at such an odd hour. The answer was soon obvious. It is all about passion. Passion to make us healthier, a passion for curbing our lifestyle-inflicted illnesses, and a passion to prevent us from ending up as patients under Stig's or his successors' knife. It is urgent! It is so pressing that Stig believed an 8 a.m. meeting on a Saturday morning was completely reasonable.

So who is this Stig? He is a professor who practiced surgery at the University of Lund in Sweden. He headed the surgery department at the university hospital for thirty years and led so many important surgical assignments both in Sweden and abroad that his CV would need all the space meant for this foreword and more. The medical database Pubmed contains more than five hundred scientific papers by Stig Bengmark, and he has tutored hundreds of doctoral candidates and other students. This shows tremendous productivity. Stig's name still has a somewhat legendary ring to it in the world of surgery; he is known for his exactitude and for his breakthrough ideas, methods, and forward thinking that have had great impact.

But who is he really? For the answer we need to look at his passion and inquisitiveness. After specializing for many years on the liver—the body's detoxifier—Stig started to question if there wasn't a way to prevent some of the serious illnesses he saw in his everyday workload. But how? Were there areas of our lifestyles that we needed to change?

When retirement gave Stig time on his hands, he decided to follow what has now been his lodestar for the last twenty-five years. He searched for the answer to why so many people develop diabetes, obesity, hypertension, heart, and circulatory problems—not to mention why there are so many digestive problems. At last he had the time to study all the medical literature and make a compilation of all that we currently know on the subject. Having decided his path, Stig accepted a position as visiting professor in London and got to work.

Soon Stig arrived at a number of conclusions that are now summarized in his twelve commandments (which you will find in this book). A new system of knowledge grew in which microbiome, dietary fiber, sugar, and how often we eat are taken very seriously. The right, "good" kind of fat has been shown not to be dangerous. Sugar ended up in the crosshairs. Stig explains how to reduce a kind of inflammation that is so low-grade we don't even know it is there; but because it is chronic, it helps to hasten aging of body tissues.

Stig tested hundreds of bacterial strains to find the ones that could best control this low-grade inflammation. This led to the introduction of several new products on the market. Suddenly he wasn't just a physician, researcher, and professor, but also an entrepreneur with a social conscience. His goal was to help us all live healthier.

Today we talk about social entrepreneurship. Perhaps this took hold in Stig long before it became a buzzword? Perhaps Stig truly is Sweden's first social entrepreneur? He is, in my opinion, one of the best social entrepreneurs; because to work to radically improve people's health is a journey toward the finest goal we can set—a healthier life.

I have to admit Stig has infected me with his passion. What started out as a collection of research collaborations has grown into something that affects my daily life. I'd rather go out to the vegetable patch than to the granary and Stig's cocktail is a daily beverage. My sugar and meat consumption is moderate. Has this improved my health? I'm not sure, but I do believe my body likes it. As I'm a scientist by profession; I can't help using myself as a guinea pig. My blood vessels show—using two different methods of measurement—forty-two years old, while my passport says sixty years old. I must admit to a bit of excess weight, but my blood fats and blood pressure are like a teenager's. This was not the case with my father at my age. He had just been hospitalized with a massively enlarged heart and very aged blood vessels.

Do I owe my results to Stig's recommendations? It is difficult to be certain when the health of one person looks anecdotal. Nevertheless, what Stig has done in several wide-ranging scientific overviews is to summarize the known literature, and use this together with his own research to draw his conclusions. Stig has translated science to the benefit of us all.

There is, of course, much more to discover and Stig doesn't hold the answers to all questions. He might, perhaps, even be wrong sometimes in his eagerness to understand. Perhaps Stig's conclusions drawn from current knowledge about how to change lifestyle for a healthier life won't stand the test of time. Personally, though, I doubt that we can get a better and more accessible summary than Stig's of today's knowledge about lifestyle and health issues. This gives Stig probably his finest title—people educator!

You who read this are lucky. You are allowed to partake of a life's work of passion. Hopefully you will be infected, just like I am, by Stig's passion!

Stockholm, October 2018
Martin Schalling, Professor of Medical Genetics,
Karolinska Institutet

Introduction

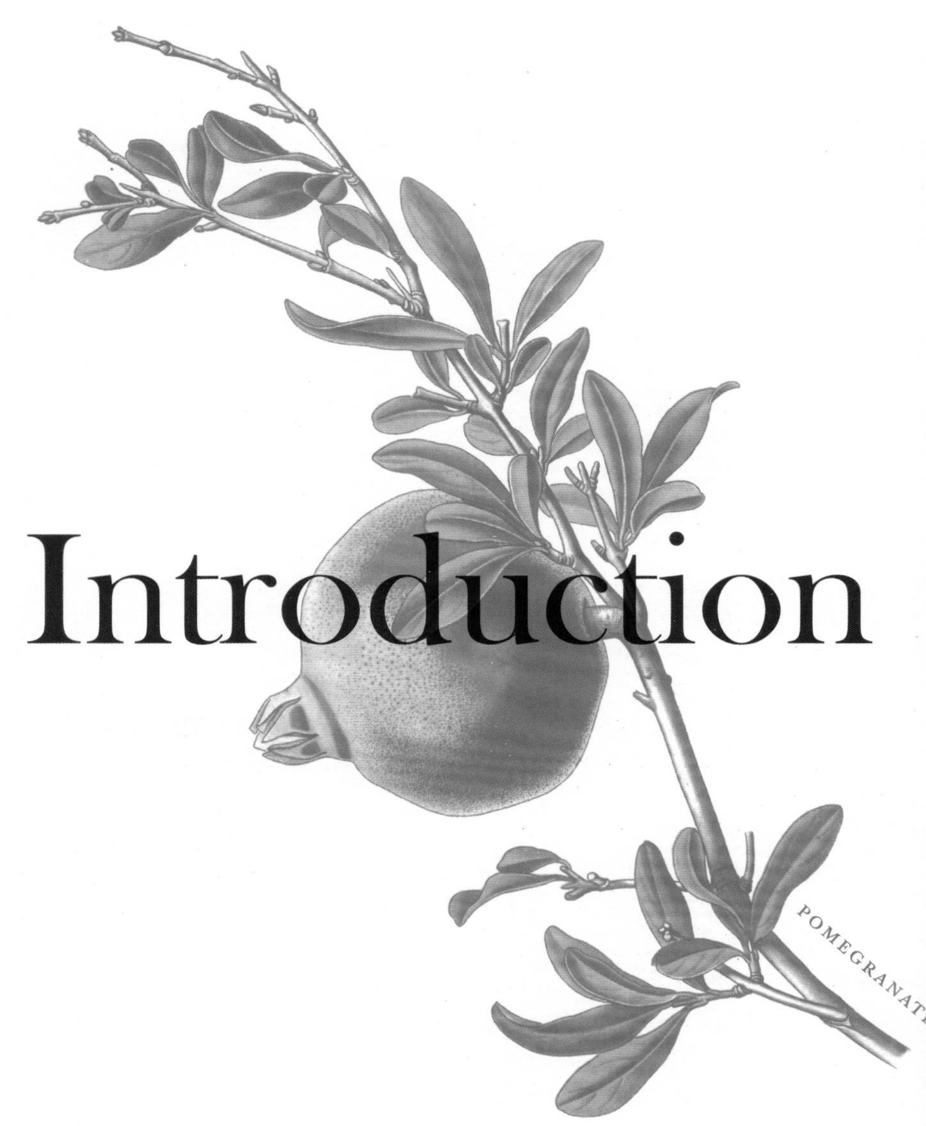

My name is Stig Bengmark.

I was born in Östervåla, outside Uppsala, Sweden, in 1929. My parents practiced a very healthy lifestyle. My father, a landscape gardener who was also a Free Church pastor, taught us the benefits and wholesomeness of the plant world.

My mother fed me lots of mashed vegetables and fruit when I was very young. In those days there weren't a lot of packaged baby cereals or canned baby foods around to stuff children with. I increasingly realize what a great gift my mother's food must have been for my intestinal flora.

My childhood experience may partially explain why I today hold forth on the subject that people ought to eat themselves healthy instead of sick. In addition, they ought to be more physically active and less stressed.

As a possible profession, I first considered psychology; perhaps psychiatry. But my impatience got the better of me, and I decided on surgery instead. I wanted to see results fast.

My thirty years as a surgeon (1958–1988) and head of surgery at the University of Lund, Sweden (1970–1994), have certainly increased my insight into human nature as well as the fragility of the human body. Despite all precautions taken, far too many patients suffered grave infections after having surgery. They fell ill even though everybody was treated with antibiotics, the miracle drug of the era.

I came to another important insight in 1986; the fact that antibiotics could do more harm than good when used in connection with surgery. You'll soon find out how I came to that realization, but from that day on, my research has concentrated on the role of the colon's good bacteria in people's health.

With time I became increasingly convinced that our bad dietary habits were at the base of our lifestyle illnesses, such as cancer, diabetes, cardiovascular disease, and Alzheimer's disease. It was evident the ghostlike connections between chronic inflammation and chronic illness tended to trigger others to follow.

Retirement, together with my position as Professor Emeritus, let me go fully into my research of intestinal flora. As of 1999 I held an unpaid honorary professorship at the University of London.

Bit by bit, my health program started to take form—an opposition to the sugar- and fat-fixated Western eating habit that is now also taking over the rest of the world.

A few years before retiring, I initiated a research effort into the production of probiotics (i.e., nutritional supplements in the form of live bacteria). The reason for this was that many people have an intestinal flora that needs to be reestablished after long and often unconscious maltreatment—before the colon could cope with a healthier diet. The result of this research was the popular beverage Proviva, which is still available in stores. Probiotics have become a recognized supplement—except where they are stopped by a healthcare system that favors pharmaceutical treatments.

Today, I can proudly say my synbiotic product has brought interest in probiotics to a wider audience. We are no longer searching for the good bacteria in the colon. In the worst-case scenario, they fled several generations ago. Instead we searched and found them in nature.

With this book I want to summarize my research to date and my method.

The young authors Lina Nerby Aurell and Mia Clase have already paved the way for the popularity of my ideas through their book *Food Pharmacy*. They have given immense attention to my extensive research and to the principal foundation of colon-friendly dietary habits.

More and more people are beginning to pay attention to the importance of the microbiota (i.e., the intestinal flora). The readership of my media outlets, which counts in the hundreds of thousands of people, provides daily proof of this, especially those who have sorted out their health problems thanks to synbiotics.

There is a stream of new books about more mindful caring for colon health. I recently saw someone summing it up as the "microbiotic revolution." In the United States they have made it more accessible to everybody by starting to talk about colon makeup. It pleases me to no end!

One thing does bother me, however. Far too many within Western healthcare systems still don't want to embrace what the new insights demand: more preventive care and more focus on lifestyle change in the fight against the skyrocketing national diseases.

As long as we don't have a supporting preventive healthcare system worth its name, I sincerely hope that you, my reader, grab the initiative yourself and choose health!

If you are pregnant, you can, through conscious lifestyle and dietary habits, immensely improve the future conditions of your child.

Whoever you are, you have the ability, through a microbiome-friendly diet, to affect your own, your family's, and your friends' dietary habits in a positive way. Can you imagine a better gift to someone you love?

Dear reader, except for a substantial reorganization of your daily diet, what will my advice cost you? A super powerful mixer! It will, however, pay for itself in no time. You can make sure of a healthier and longer life through this change of lifestyle.

Take a look and get inspiration from my dear wife Marianne's recipe collection.

The path is laid out. Welcome!

Höganäs and London, November 2018
Stig Bengmark

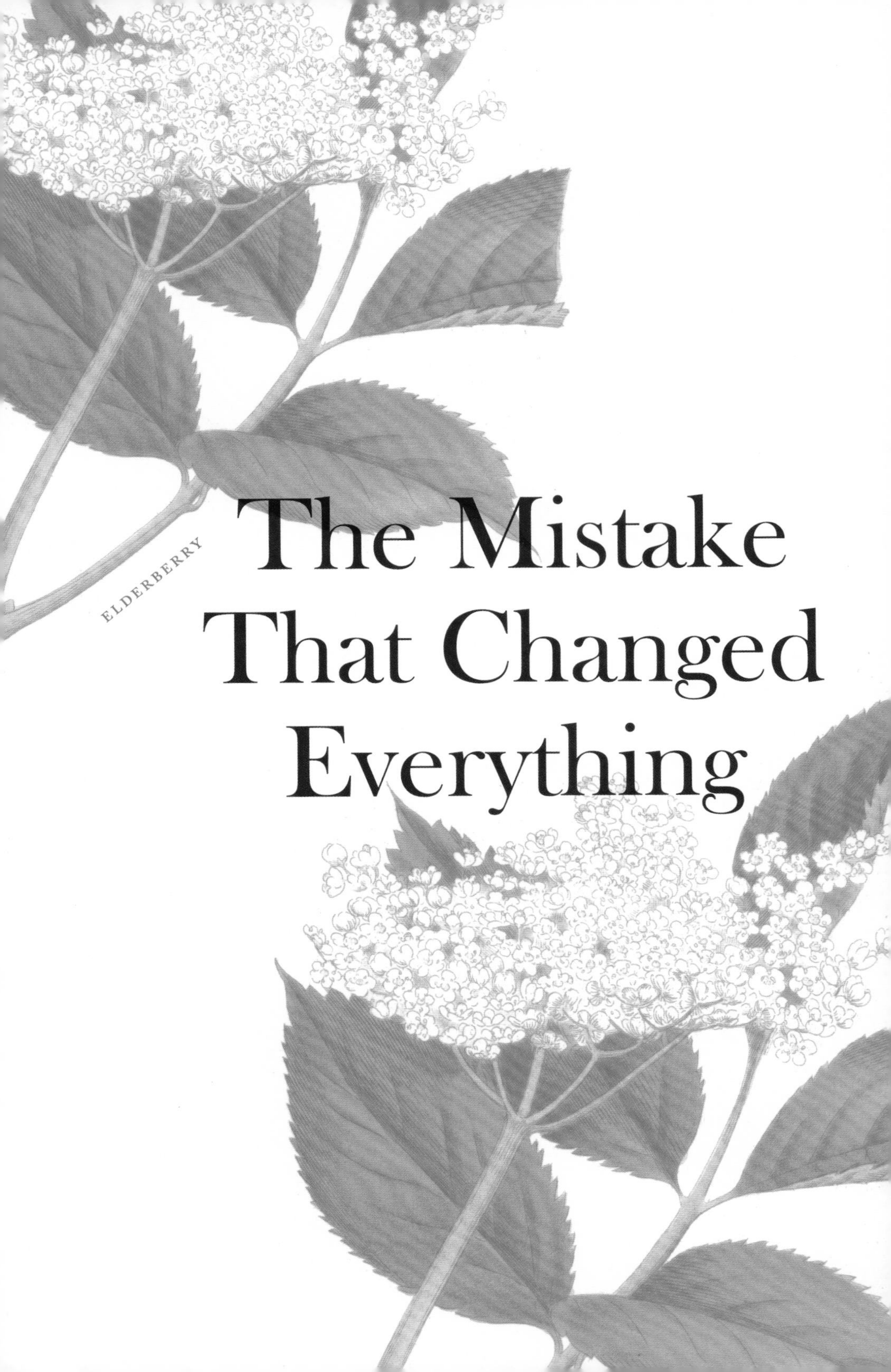

The Mistake That Changed Everything

01

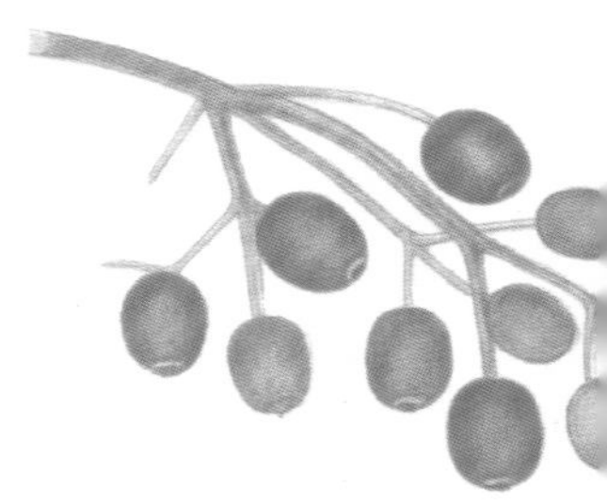

A mistake made in my surgery clinic in the 1990s gave me new and amazing insights into how intestinal bacteria affect our health.

I decided to look deeper into questions about intestinal bacteria and digestion. Our Western dietary habits proved to be even more destructive than I had imagined. My life's project increasingly turned into a wide-ranging education issue. I wanted to give as many people as possible the chance to eat themselves healthy.

The first two chapters must unfortunately be somber and focused on the biggest threats to intestinal health in our opulent society. However, the rest of the book is all about how easily you can change your dietary habits and improve your health immensely!

I WORKED AS a surgeon until I retired. As one of the pioneers in extensive abdominal surgery, my specialty was the major organs such as the liver and the pancreas. When cancer was present, we usually removed the entire pancreas or up to 75 percent of the liver.

Even though the surgery was successful, the recuperation wasn't always to my satisfaction. Serious infections often occurred. It bothered me to no end that I could not promise a guaranteed success for the surgical procedure I prescribed for my patients. All too often I had to cancel a vacation or a trip abroad because a patient upon whom I had operated suddenly turned critical.

Bad News . . . and Good

One day a new perspective on the problem arrived like a gift from above.

I had asked the young physician Henrik Ekberg, later a professor of organ transplantation (1951–2012), to study in depth our latest eighty-one major liver surgeries. Suddenly, he knocked on my door and said he had both bad and good news.

What he told me frightened me terribly. He said in a number of cases they had *forgotten* to administer antibiotics. By the standard operating procedure of the time, antibiotics were to be given a few days before and then during seven to ten days after surgery.

Shock and horror! How was this possible? Isn't our university clinic meant to be a role model for other hospitals in the country? Deeply shocked, I sank down into my chair, and Ekberg added, "But, Stig—wait, I said I have good news, too! *All infections were in patients who had been administered antibiotics!* There were no infections at all in the patients who had not been given any antibiotics."

This changed everything. Could the antibiotics have killed off the beneficial intestinal flora?

During my last years as surgeon, observations of my own and others pointed toward a correlation between infectious complications, intestinal flora/colon function, and the patient's own immune defense. Strengthened by Ekberg's confirmatory revelation, I was now eager to further research the intestinal flora.

Emeritus—A Sense of Freedom!

For decades, society has expected researchers, like the clergy, to work until the very end. They are not pensioned off, they are just released from administrative drudgery and are called *Emeritus*. There are expectations from both the employer and the emeritus that the emerita/emeritus will continue to spread their knowledge during the coming years, to the best of their ability.

My hope is that this book—an example of a twenty-five-year span of emeritus work—will contribute to the continuation of this splendid tradition.

In 1994, I became Professor Emeritus at the medical faculty in Lund, Sweden. I then looked forward to extending my knowledge about disease, especially chronic diseases and their causes. Our present-day society is staggering under the weight of the fast-growing and soon unsupportable cost of public healthcare.

I wanted to be able to point at nutrition's important role in preventive medicine, and eventually convince the healthcare system to accept its part of the responsibility. My conviction was, with increased care taken of the intestinal flora, we would dramatically reduce instances of illness. Thus, we would reduce society's cost for healthcare.

When the time for emeritus neared, several foreign universities approached me with offers to take my future research to their facilities as an honorary visiting professor. The big deal is that you can then use university resources and collaborate with and inspire other scientists who are often visiting researchers and doctoral candidates from the world over. London was my choice, and since 1999/2000, I've had the privilege to do my work at the University of London.

A scientific investigation by the Norwegian professor of immunology Per Brandzaeg, showing that 70 percent to 80 percent of the immune system is situated in the colon, inspired me to continue my research. According to Per Brandzaeg, the major part of immunoglobulin is formed in the colon; it strengthens the immune response in the body and also contributes to training immune cells to perform their task.

Health Is Situated in a Healthy Colon and the Immune System

As a new Emeritus, I used all the time at my disposal to read about our national diseases. It has become more and more evident to me that there are similar—perhaps even the same—mechanisms leading to the development of these diseases.

Unfortunately, we don't know why one person will develop cancer and another MS (multiple sclerosis). What we do know is the person who has developed one chronic condition is at a significantly higher risk of developing two, three, or several more during their lifetime. *Clustering*, as this phenomenon is called, is well worth studying and preventing. Too few of the affected have the stamina or can be persuaded to make any changes at all to improve their lifestyle.

At about that time many became aware that antibiotics hadn't shown the positive effect hoped for. My focus then became taking a closer look at the importance of *nutrition*, which is also very much about how the body's immune system functions.

After extensive studies, it was evident to me that the development of chronic disease depends on prolonged activation of the body's defense mechanism when it is exposed to psychological and/or physical stress. This phenomenon is well known as acute stress, APR* (acute phase response). However, as an association with prolonged and permanent chronic disease, the phenomenon was completely unexplored. I wrote an article about this and suggested that it ought to be called CPR (chronic phase response) in that connection. Reactions like APR and CPR are basically acute and chronically elevated inflammation.

Today, it is commonly accepted that "inflammation is the mother of disease." Scientific studies on animals and humans have shown people with chronic illness often have lost a large part of their beneficial intestinal flora. It has been partially replaced with harmful bacteria carrying with them all the negative consequences for our health.

Dysbiosis always exists, for example, in obese persons and persons suffering from hypertension. This is shown by a significant

* 248–253.

reduction of beneficial bacteria content (*diversity*), as well as in the total amount of certain important bacteria strains (*richness*).

Two kinds of bacteria have received a lot of attention and show perfectly how risky behavior can negatively affect the intestines. One is the *Firmicutes*, which dominate the microbiota when someone eats an excess of sugary and fatty foods. The other is *Bacteroidetes*, which dominate the microbiota the more unprocessed and fiber-rich someone's diet is.

For example, patients with obesity and hypertension have shown to have a very limited set of beneficial bacteria varieties, and a very limited amount of bacteria in total. This strongly reduces the release of short-chain fatty acids in the intestine, such as acetic acid and butyric acid; products that are imperative for preserving intestinal impermeability and the immune system's optimal function.

I want you to get acquainted here with three phenomena within the nutritional supplements field that you will meet up with. All have the purpose to enrich the intestinal flora.

Prebiotics means, literally, "before life." They are fibers (complex carbohydrates) that feed the intestinal flora. Probiotics are live bacteria that enrich the colon and have a positive effect on health. Synbiotics stands for a blend of live bacteria and dietary fiber. It is a solution I have developed and will revisit later in the book.

Rush to Reevaluate Antibiotics

Early in the process I took the initiative for a project that became Probi, a Swedish publicly listed biotechnical company that develops probiotics and sells, for example, the product Proviva.

It is a question of changing our perception of antibiotics and, above all, our perception of beneficial bacteria. As a physician and researcher I experienced this as something very urgent. Even today, lo and behold, antibiotics are still being casually handed out after surgery, even though study after study has shown them having negative effects or causing negative outcomes. Even today, about every third patient experiences infections after major abdominal surgery. For liver transplant, the number is actually more like every second.

In 1999 I started a project together with some research colleagues in which we collected a little over five hundred different lactic acid bacteria. As I had spent years researching the reason for chronic disease and realized that inflammation was an important component, our goal was to find an elite group of anti-inflammatory bacteria. Special interest was given to the bacteria's ability to strengthen each other's anti-inflammatory properties.

> "It is indisputable today that the intestinal flora's composition has strong bearing on our health."

Based on our studies we chose and took out patents on eight specific lactic acid bacteria. Because we established early on that the bacteria could multiply in the colon with the help of dietary fiber, we combined the bacteria with a "packed lunch" of four different plant fibers, known as particularly good food for bacteria. This became the first synbioticum!

Early animal testing showed the combination's unique characteristics in decreasing inflammation and protecting the body's tissues against injury.

We have now, for nearly twenty years worldwide, studied everything from IBS (irritable bowel syndrome) to cancer patients and liver transplant recipients. Time after time the synbiotic has shown itself successful in building up the intestinal flora and strengthening the immune system in seriously ill patients, especially in the ICU. Up until now, our focus has been on infections and inflammations. However, lately we have even focused on the contribution to the immune system and to reducing the risk for chronic illnesses by adding our good bacteria and fiber daily.

Today it is indisputable that the intestinal flora's composition has a strong connection to our health.

Disease Patterns Through the Ages

Our forebears had approximately one malign bacterium among a million good ones. It is not at all unusual that the bad bacteria take over and dominate the intestinal flora with today's dietary habits, stress, lack of exercise, and our consumption of antibiotics and other pharmaceuticals.

The disease picture is shown to change sharply over time. In the nineteenth century, infectious and parasite-related diseases dominated; tuberculosis/lung disease and STDs featured prominently.

After 1880, cancer as well as cardiovascular and lung disease as registered illnesses have increased in northern Europe from 20 percent to over 70 percent, and chronic illness continued to increase fast.

During the twentieth century diseases such as cancer, diabetes, Alzheimer's disease, and cardiovascular disease spread more and more across the Western world. They are sometimes referred to by an umbrella term, diseases of affluence (NCD—noncommunicable disease), because they seem to relate to improved living conditions in the prosperous Western world. Perhaps the main problem with this lifestyle is quite simply dietary excess.

It is predicted that the "affluenza diseases" are going to double in less time than our human life span because earlier developing countries have now adopted what was called a Westernized lifestyle.

A tsunami of chronic illness has its epicenter in the southern United States. States such as Alabama, Louisiana, and Mississippi are the leaders. However, they are looking to lose the leader shirt to the Near East, the Arab world, India, and surprisingly certain African nations. Obesity and hypertension, often the earliest signs of an illness-inducing lifestyle, are acknowledged more openly nowadays as the forerunners to chronic illness. It's estimated that 75 percent of the earth's population that suffers from hypertension lives in Africa, where every third person suffers from hypertension.

In conclusion, diabetes will have doubled in 2050 while Alzheimer's disease and cancer will have tripled in Western countries like Great Britain and United States.

The Price We Pay for Our Industrialized Household

A large part of the changing disease specter can be explained thus: The transformation from a natural household to an industrial household has come at a high price.

Our Stone Age forebears ate more than five hundred different, often fresh and raw, plants yearly. Food to be saved was dug down and covered with earth or dried. Both ways produced fermentation, which meant that the food acquired lots of beneficial lactobacilli. Our Stone Age ancestors taught us how to prepare sauerkraut and sourdough, brew beer, and make wine.

Today our Western population takes its nutrition from a very narrow sample. Eighty percent of today's diet comes from seventeen plants and 50 percent from eight different kinds of grain. In addition, the food is heated, dried, irradiated, and packaged. The plants used are usually inferior from the very beginning and contain large amounts of sugar. This is well known to reduce nutrients dramatically, especially antioxidants.

We can learn a lot from the Japanese example! As a group, the Japanese have changed their lifestyle dramatically after World War II. The population's changeover from self-catering household to industrial processed food was incredibly stark. For example, the intake of eggs increased nine times, meat twelve times, and dairy products twenty times.

What happened? During the first fifty years Japan registered a twenty-five-fold increase in chronic illnesses such as breast and prostate cancer.

ANCESTRAL CALORIE CONSUMPTION

	Abchazien S. Caucausus, Georgia	Vilcabamba (Ecuador)	Henza (Japan)
% calories from carbohydrates	69 %	74 %	71 %
% calories from fat	18 %	15 %	17 %
% calories from protein	13 %	11 %	10 %
Total daily calorie intake	1 800	1 700	1 800
% plants in food	90 %	99 %	99 %
% animal foods	10 %	1 %	1 %
Sugar consumption	0	0	0
Processed foods consumption	0	0	0
Incidence of obesity	0	0	0

Our Microbiome Is in Crisis—Our Healthcare Is Powerless

Many conditions appear today that were unknown for the medical profession in the past. The healthcare system has been totally surprised by this, and because of the lack of knowledge, these problems have not always been seen as serious. Due to this, there is still a considerable deficiency of effective methods to counteract and to treat these problems.

The list shows the common conditions likely to constitute a larger part of our millennium's healthcare headache. In parallel, we will also suffer from the effects of a mindless and exaggerated use of pharmaceuticals. Specifically, our uncritical use of antibiotics will characterize our era's medical practice.

The prognosis for 2050 is that resistant bacteria will be the leading cause of death worldwide—more common than cancer.

Do study the percentages in the table below! It is dizzying how quickly the diseases have increased in less than thirty years and alarming our healthcare system in many cases still doesn't know how to treat these illnesses properly.

Chronic fatigue syndrome	11,027%
Bipolar disorder in children and teens	10,833%
Fibromyalgia	7,727%
Autism	2,094%
ADHD	819%
Lupus	787%
Hypothyroid	702%
Osteoarthritis	449%
Sleep apnea	430%
Alzheimer's disease	299%
Depression	80%
Asthma	142%

Vast Ignorance Concerning the Potential of Bacteria

Our microbiome and our immune system are the object of an ongoing, if slow, deterioration. A strong reason is the increasing consumption of processed food following a decrease of plant fiber and plant antioxidants.

Research shows that the Western population has lost, overall, about half of the good gut bacteria that our ancestors possessed, while populations living more like our ancestors have, more or less, managed to retain theirs.

Perhaps a contributing factor is that today's caregivers are schooled in *chemical/pharmaceutical medicine*, which is in sharp contrast to earlier times' biological focus.

The knowledge necessary to use living organisms to treat illness is lacking in chemical medicine. Chemical medicine, therefore, has been ignorant of the gut flora's/microbiota's importance for our health.

The crux of adding bacteria and plant ingredients to food is oddly still unknown today.

Too Few Vegetables, Too Much Heating

It is important to remember that our beneficial gut bacteria are dependent on a steady and extensive supply of plants in amazingly large quantities. If this is absent, the good bacteria will pack their bags and leave. We need to take that into consideration daily.

While the researchers have tried to follow this, many attempts have been made to map the kind of food our ancestors ate—and to reintroduce the same. They have had limited success. Nevertheless, it is calculated that each day our ancestors ate between 1¼ and 3¼ pounds (1–1½ kg) fresh and uncooked plant foods, containing at least 5¼ ounces (150 g) of plant fiber. Health authorities in the Western world recommend at least 1¼ ounces daily (35 g). The depressing truth is that the average consumption in our part of the world is only around ½ ounce (15 g) a day. More current studies have shown that we need about 1¼ to 3¼ lbs (1–1½ kg) of fresh, raw, or frozen plant matter daily to stay healthy, even if we can see important improvement with 1¾ pounds (800 g) daily. How this intake of plant food can reduce the risk for different illnesses is evident in the list below.

A DAILY CONSUMPTION OF 1¾ POUNDS (800 G) OF FRUIT AND VEGETABLES IS ASSOCIATED WITH:

- 28 percent reduced risk for cardiovascular disease
- 24 percent reduced risk for heart disease
- 33 percent reduced risk for stroke
- 13 percent reduced risk for cancer (all)
- 31 percent reduced risk for premature death

How do we benefit from food compared to our ancestors? The simple answer is that Stone Age people ate themselves to healthy gut flora while today's very inferior dietary habits give us a much poorer immunity.

THE SHORTCUT

Approximately 60 percent: Sugar and sugar-like substances enter the upper portion of the small intestine, primarily through the blood.

(During the Stone Age: <15 percent)

THE SLOWER ROUTE

Approximately 30 percent: Animal and vegetable fats enter the body by the lymphatic system and circulate during several hours.

(During the Stone Age: <10 percent)

THE HEALTHY ROUTE

Less than 20 percent: Raw vegetables and fruit is nutrition for the microbiome and reach the colon after two to three hours. They strengthen the immune system and prevent inflammation.

(During the Stone Age plant matter was the main part of the diet, approx. 80 percent)

Many important nutrients are destroyed if the food is prepared using high heat: roasting, grilling, frying, or baking at high temperatures. Today's highly processed food is taken up in the small intestine and becomes an unacceptable burden on the interior organs, primarily on the liver and pancreas. Heating contributes to the postprandial inflammation that Westerners suffer from. We see excessive increase of the bacterial endotoxin in blood circulation and the whole body, which is a recent discovery. High levels of endotoxins in tissues and blood are a recurrent factor in many chronic illnesses.

Obesity—a Sure Sign of Excess Consumption

Jon Brower Minnoch (1941–1983) lived in the United States and was forty-two years old when he died. Jon's weight was approximated to 1,400 pounds (635 kg), and he was the fattest person in history. He committed, like millions with him in the Western world, a state-sponsored "suicide" with knife and fork. This was completely possible with the help of cheap, refined, and calorie-laden farm produce.

His life was miserable, and his care cost the community a small fortune. This is an all-too-common problem in the Western world.

Recently, it was reported in Great Britain the direct cost for treating obese patients has increased 350 percent during the last five years. This is enormously troubling in a country where the national health system is in an economic crisis.

Obesity arrived with the advent of industrial farming and has increased in step with industrial farming's development and more refined products. The worldwide tsunami of chronic illnesses mentioned earlier also geographically follows the highly forced farming development.

Postprandial Inflammation and Toxic Distribution

Each meal, regardless of amount or content, illustrates how the levels of sugar, fat, and bacterial toxins increase in the blood. This affects all organs, not least the heart and brain. The glucose level stays usually elevated for an hour, and the level of endotoxins a bit longer, around 1½ hours.

The fat level, unfortunately, stays elevated for around four hours. Consequently this means that many walk around with elevated blood-fat levels all day. A lot of Westerners probably suffer from postprandial inflammation during the better part of the day.

This problem is, of course, worsened the more we add sugar, fat, and endotoxin-laden foods that elevate these levels in the body.

The larger the part of processed foods, as well as of sugar and long-chain fatty acids (animal fats and vegetable/seed oils, even olive oil), the bigger and more long-lasting is the postprandial inflammation. The problem with long-chain fatty acids is that they can only be absorbed by the lymphatic system. The process works through small fat globules that spread from the intestine by the lymph, which then empties into the blood circulation. These fat globules act like a form of Trojan horse: they "smuggle" in colon bacteria, bacterial remnants, and bacterial toxins like endotoxins into the body.

The grade of inflammation that an inferior Western diet can produce is estimated to equal what you'll see after a person has quickly smoked three cigarettes. The picture describes the changes that have been observed in endotoxins in connection with ingestion of a standard meal.

> "The level of inflammation a Western dietary meal can provoke is estimated to correspond to what is seen after a person has quickly smoked three cigarettes."

Hundreds of toxins that the malign colon bacteria produce have been identified.

This can create serious problems if the kidneys are not functioning optimally. The majority, but not all, can today be resolved temporarily via dialysis.

When using the older method, hemodialysis, the toxins become especially problematic. As the kidneys normally try to eliminate toxins immediately as they enter the body, and this kind of dialysis is only performed a few times per week, the level of toxins have time to get particularly elevated, not least the endotoxins.

However, fewer patients need to go through the strenuous, with toxic side effects, hemodialysis today. The newer dialysis method

ELEVATION OF BACTERIAL TOXIN ENDOTOXIN AFTER A STANDARD MEAL

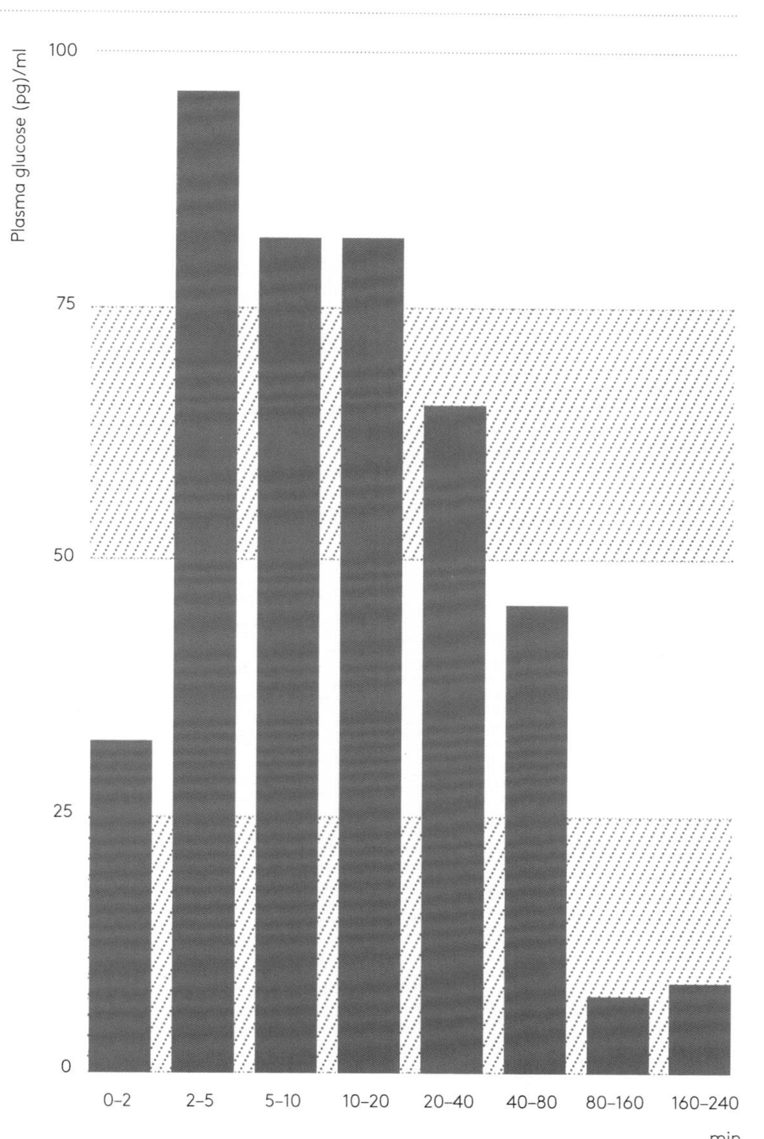

(peritoneal dialysis) lets the patient do the cleaning at home in a simple and less uncomfortable way by filtering fluid and replacing it with clean fluid four times a day.

Affect Your Health Resources!

The first chapters in this book might seem pessimistic and demanding. Just imagine what a wide unconsciousness exists in our so-called enlightened era! So many negative effects that might happen when toxins and malign bacteria start to invade a person's intestinal flora! Counteracting the degradation of your intestinal system also demands willingness and patience. But believe me: it is easy to follow my method to combat bad gut flora! The rest of the book is filled with uncomplicated advice and tips and several of my wife Marianne's favorite recipes.

The reason I explain how chronic illness occurs is so you can learn how to avoid this happening. Your reward can be that the illness, which often follows inflammation, might never happen. This is my optimistic view of your chance for good health: You control approximately 70 percent of your health resources. Lifestyle changes, even later in life, reduce illness frequency by at least 50 percent and prolong life considerably.

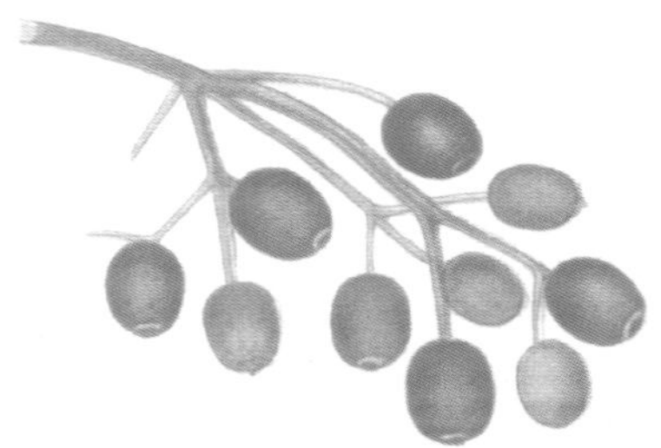

Avoid the Chronic Illness Trap!

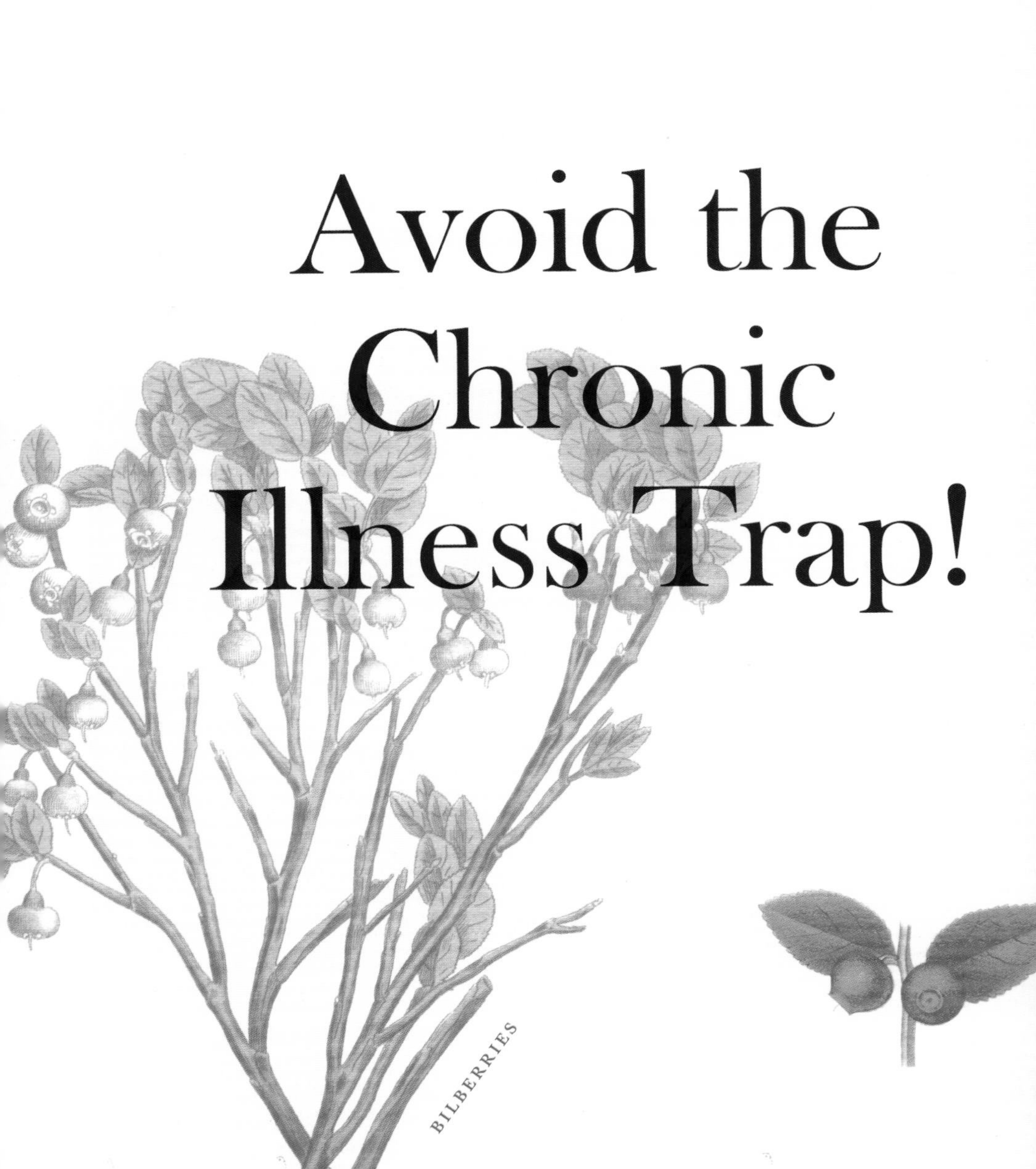

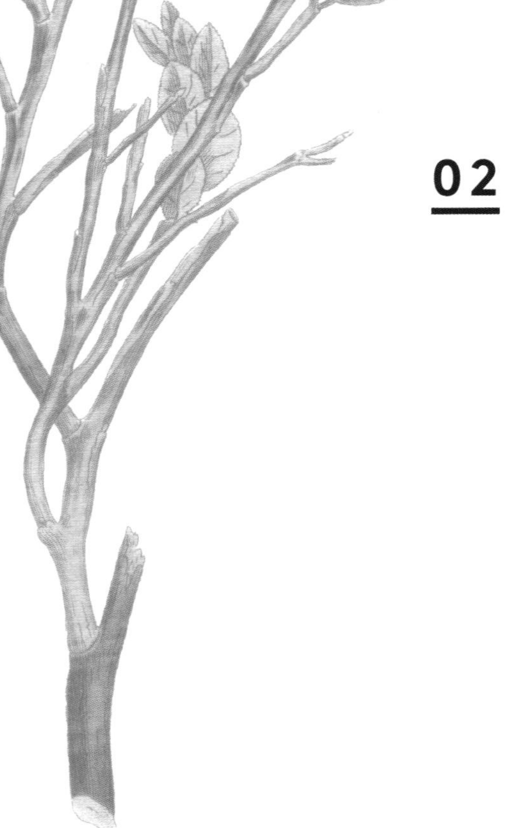

02

A few years ago I set aside a whole working year to get a better understanding of chronic illness. To my surprise, many of my earlier impressions proved to be right: everything stemmed from the same root cause! All of these illnesses are siblings or at least cousins.

Here we delve deeper into the connections between chronic inflammation and chronic illness so you can learn how to avoid them.

MANY, IF NOT all, chronic illnesses are the result of the lengthy defense reaction and an exhaustion of the immune system that chronic inflammation creates.

There are many ways you yourself can combat this. But to do this you need knowledge.

"Inflammatio" Means Fire

Inflammation has been known as a concept for hundreds of years. The word origin is Latin: *inflammatio* means fire. The word was originally used to describe changes appearing in body tissue when some form of injury or infection threatens it.

Inflammation's five characteristics were described early on as: redness (rubor), swelling (tumor), pain (dolor), locally increased heat (calor), and reduced function (functio laesa). Several of these reactions are the effects of the body's mobilization against an injury and its wish to start the healing process.

We have long known the importance of white blood cells in this process. As soon as there is an injury, white blood cells leave the blood circulation as soon as possible to surround the injury/ infection and to stop its spread; at the same time they destroy/ eat the bacteria and the rest of the injured cells—a reaction called *phagocytos*. However, today we know the process is much more complex than this. The reaction is now called acute phase reaction (i.e., the immediate inflammatory response). Following this response there are often tissue injuries such as scar tissue formation and organ adhesions.

What Is Chronic Inflammation?

We recognize that, nowadays, chronic inflammation is a commonly occurring state for many of us.

In contrast to the acute phase reaction already mentioned, chronic inflammation is particularly discreet and often very difficult to identify.

Low-key signs might be: unexplained fatigue, sleep disturbances, headache, alopecia, early graying of hair, dandruff, acne, unexplained cutaneous eruptions and redness, dry eye, brittle nails, dry mouth or excessive saliva production, reduced sex drive, irregular menstruation, unexplained chronic constipation or diarrhea, osteoporosis of unknown origin, frequent unexplained infections and influenza, frequent depressive episodes, unexplained breathlessness, sweaty feet and palms, etc.

Many illnesses that start in early childhood, such as allergies and ADHD, also show significant chronic inflammation.

"Chronic inflammation is particularly discreet and often very difficult to identify."

The inflammatory strain put on the body by chronic inflammation also makes the ill person's body more susceptible to attacks from a second or third illness. It's not uncommon that illnesses such as Alzheimer's disease, diabetes, and cancer appear after several years.

We haven't managed to find the answer yet to the question as to why the disease course may start with cancer in one individual, diabetes in another, and Alzheimer's disease in a third.

Medication Is Not the Answer

There are thousands, probably tens of thousands, of factors contributing to the development of chronic inflammation. We are, for the most part, not at all talking about inherited, genetic traits.

Contributing factors can be anything from the environment of your grandfather's birth and childhood; your mother's lifestyle before and during her pregnancy, and also during the time you were breastfed (the period when the immune system is programmed and calibrated)—up to your own lifestyle. It's considered that a "bad" lifestyle inheritance contributes about 5 percent to the risk for chronic illness later in life. A mother's inferior lifestyle before, during, and after the pregnancy contributes a further 20–25 percent to the health of the baby and has long-term effects.

It's not unusual that persons with above-mentioned complaints look to their physicians for help, usually resulting in a prescription for some kind of pharmaceutical. Unfortunately, pharmaceuticals don't help in the majority of inflammation cases but instead result in further prescriptions of one or more medications.

As you have already understood, my opinion is that a lifestyle change is more effective than an increase in pharmaceutical prescriptions. To me the connection is clear: chronic inflammation is the result of us abandoning our ancestors' life and dietary styles.

It Starts in the Colon— Self-Evident Through the Ages

It is vital for good digestive health that the colon is allowed to work the way it was designed to. The problem with today's Western diet is that the digestive system's vital work has been sidelined.

All the food we eat will sooner or later leave the intestines, some of it entering the bloodstream for transport to the body's cells. So far, so good. Now the question is: Where does the uptake of food occur—in the small intestine, or in the colon three to four hours later?

The longer the food stays in the intestine, the better. It is the degree of processing the food has gone through that decides where the uptake will happen. To a certain extent, food that is preprocessed in commercial manufacturing, and then additionally in the family kitchen, can be considered "predigested." This causes the uptake of it to occur high in the small intestine, doing the body a great disservice.

> "It is always desirable that the food uptake happens far down in the colon."

The unprocessed food, whether it be raw, frozen raw, fruits, vegetables, or root vegetables, is so hard to digest it is transported for three to four hours to the colon, where it is broken down by the gut flora (microbiota). It is always desirable to have food digested far down in the colon.

AN ACTIVATED COLON HAS BEEN PAR FOR THE COURSE THROUGH MILLIONS OF YEARS.

Digestion through an active colon dominated for over millions of years. The body, in this health-promoting way, took up approximately 80 percent of the food eaten.

When unprocessed or harder-to-digest food reaches the colon, it will also feed the wide variety of benign microbiota. This also facilitates the reproduction of the good bacteria.

All this makes it possible for the microbiota to fill the vital functions necessary for optimal health.

A BENIGN MICROBIOTA'S FUNCTIONS ARE TO:

1

Suppress dominance by malignant disease-producing bacteria. If the malignant bacteria are allowed to dominate unimpeded, they'll send toxins into the body or might even enter the body themselves. They create inflammation with accompanying obesity and diverse ailments.

2

Stimulate the immune system. The largest part of the immune system is situated in the intestines. The majority of the body's immunoglobulins are produced here. In addition, the immune cells are "honed" for their functions throughout the body.

3

Release wholesome substances from the plants we eat, for example: short-chain fatty acids, amino acids, vitamins, and antioxidants. These are taken up and will benefit the body. (Antioxidants are chemical structures that counteract oxidation, a process that over time harms the cells.)

4

Bring energy to the body, glucose among other things, but at the pace it is needed (i.e., slow release) instead of the shock when refined sugar is eaten and is absorbed in great quantities high up in the small intestine.

FOR OPTIMAL UPTAKE IN THE COLON EAT ACCORDING TO THE 80/10/10 PRINCIPLE

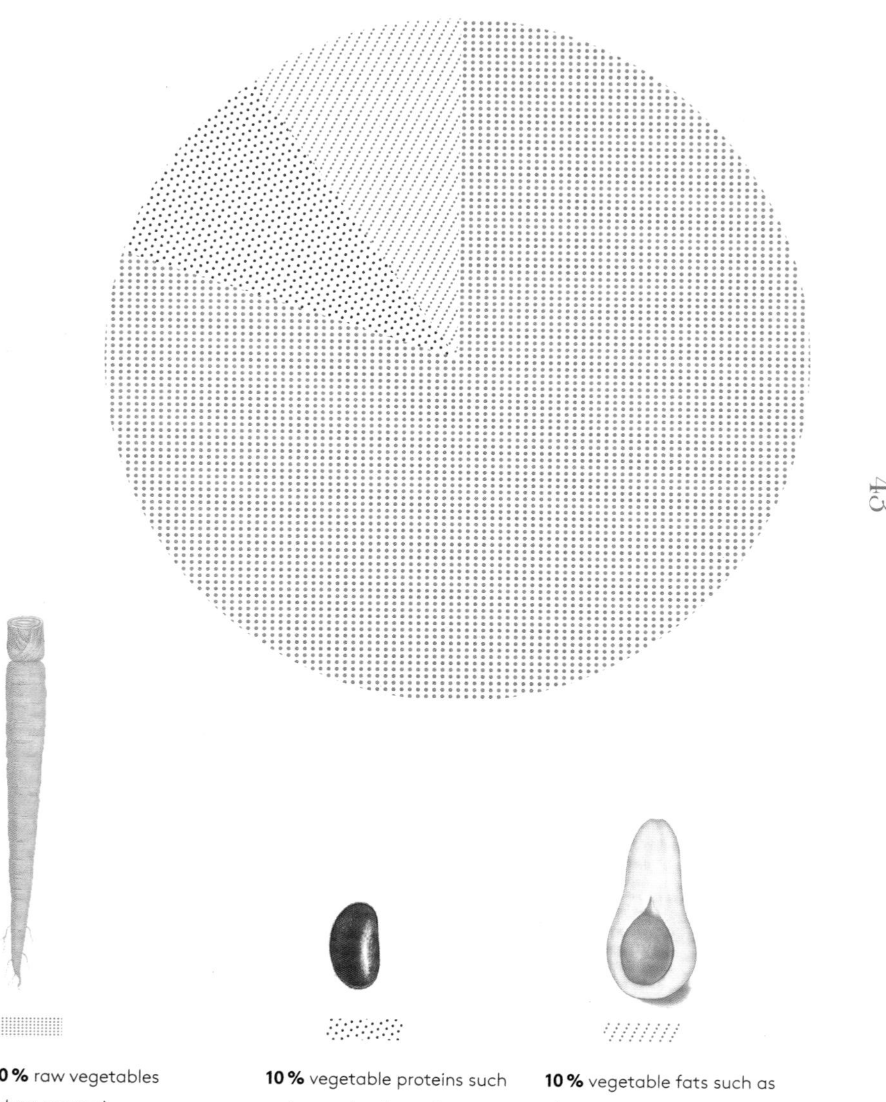

80 % raw vegetables (plant matter)

10 % vegetable proteins such as beans, lentils, and nuts and almonds

10 % vegetable fats such as olives, avocado, and coconut

Refined Foods Sneak Past

Our modern foods are absorbed high up in the small intestine because the industries, and/or we in the home kitchen, have tried to replace the work our intestinal flora has done for millions of years. While this shortcut was only taken with a fraction (less than 15%) of the food our ancestors ate, it has today become the highway for all the sugary and sugar-like foods we are consuming.

As much as 60 percent of the food we eat today is absorbed in the small intestine, losing all the health benefits we mentioned earlier.

This is in addition to many other disadvantages, which over time, become life threatening:

Our digestive organs become greatly overtaxed if forced to work to get rid of the excess glucose in the blood. The immune defense is lowered, weight might increase, and colds are more frequent.

To optimize the absorption in the colon, it is best to eat according to the 80/10/10 principle: a diet that is completely dominated by raw plants (80%) with the addition of 10 percent fatty fruits (i.e., olives, avocado, and coconut) and 10% protein-rich vegetables such as peas, beans, lentils, nuts, almonds, seeds, and similar food items.

ARE THE GREENS GOING DOWN THE DRAIN?

All too many believe that preparing "fine cuisine" means removing a lot of the exterior of vegetables and fruits when cleaning them. What does your sink look like after you've prepared leeks or beets? You likely discard a lot that could be consumed.

Humans today throw away (or feed to animals) some of the most nutritious parts of vegetables, fruit, and grains.

Not everybody realizes that nutrients in fruits and vegetables are distributed more unevenly than imagined. There is, for example, a huge difference between the root of root vegetables and their greens, where the greens show superior value: lower calorie count, lower fat and sugar content, and several times higher amounts of important minerals and vitamins.

The health benefits reaped from eating more of what grows above- than belowground emphasizes that we should prefer the root vegetables' green leaves instead of the root itself or at least retain as much as possible of the greens.

My advice to you is: don't throw away the apple core or the beet greens! Nutrients in fruits and the root vegetables are often located in the parts we don't eat—in the seeds and the cores of apples and oranges, melons and pears. For example, there is 740 percent less sugar in the beet greens than in the beet itself, and 304 percent more magnesium! So, let this wholesomeness travel on down straight to the colon. The "travel route" can, for example, go via green drinks or smoothies.

"Don't throw away the apple core or the beet greens!"

The same advice applies to our grains:

If you look closely at a grain like wheat you'll find it is composed of roughly three parts: the bran, the endosperm (flour), and the germ. Nature has provided the bran, which protects the grain from exterior attacks, with lots of fiber and antioxidants.

The germ, which is going into the ground to grow a large plant, also provides plenty of nutrients. The flour, on the other hand, which doesn't really provide any nutritional value at all, is mainly empty calories. In spite of this, through the decades humans have only kept the nonnutritious flour for themselves and given the majority of the shell/bran to the pigs to keep their digestion in working order. A lot of the germs are also sold to mink farms so the minks will grow shiny, beautiful pelts for the export market.

FEED THE PROTECTIVE BACTERIA!

While I, and many with me, fight for fiber-rich, mineral-rich, and antioxidant-rich food for our microbiota, it might be appropriate to explain how our bodies' bacterial flora function. Our bodies are crawling with microorganisms, especially bacteria. It might sound strange, but it is a fact that they are everywhere on and in us—on the skin, in the hair, in the vagina, in the digestive system, and in the respiratory system. Their proper function is vital for our health and well-being.

A human is essentially born sterile, but at the moment of birth the baby gets a touch of, thereby inheriting, the mother's bacteria. During the months following the birth, the surrounding world, and primarily the mother's milk, enriches the baby's gut flora with several kinds of bacteria. The number of protective bacteria in a healthy body then grows quickly. In principle, these bacteria stay the same throughout life. An individual's collection and pattern of protective bacteria (also called the microbiome) is so specific it would be possible to use someone's feces as a means of identification.

Unfortunately, we don't respect the nutritional needs of the microbiome as much as we would if we knew the requirements. In fact, we've done quite the opposite. We've made the microbiome's life miserable by refusing it the fiber-rich, mineral-rich, and antioxidant-rich food it wants—or, at least, we're not providing it with enough of it.

In addition, against their will, we're exposing the gut flora's beneficial bacteria to far too many different chemicals. Some of these chemicals are inherently in the foods, and others are created through preparation of food. Gluten in certain grains is one, casein in milk another, and acrylamide is one of the toxins produced through heating.

Researcher Hans Christian Gram's Insight into Bacteria

Apart from the diet itself, which can be more or less gut friendly, there is also a profound knowledge of the bacteria's fight against each other.

Nearly one hundred years ago, a Danish researcher whose last name was Gram watched how certain bacteria absorbed color through their cell walls while others didn't. Bacteria that color in a gram-coloring test are since then called Gram positives (Gram+) while the ones that don't color are called Gram negative (Gram–). The majority of Gram+ bacteria are benign while the majority of Gram– bacteria are malignant.

What's so great about Gram-positive bacteria is that, provided they like their environment, they have the capability to push away the inflammation-provoking and illness-causing gram-negative bacteria. However, Gram+ bacteria require lots of minerals, primarily magnesium, to be able to grow to dominate.

Raw, frozen, or lightly steamed kale, broccoli, spinach, red beet greens, carrots, and avocado are sure sources for feeding the good bacteria. The foods in the list below are especially rich in magnesium:

RICH IN MAGNESIUM

Pumpkin and squash seeds	540
Cacao	520
Sesame seeds	350
Almonds	280
Soybeans	265
Cashews	260
Dried rose hips	240
Oat bran	235
Peanuts	190

(Mg/3 1/2 oz) (Mg/100g)

GRAM+ SHOULD BE ALLOWED TO TAKE CHARGE AGAIN!

Apart from pushing away the malignant bacteria, Gram+ bacteria fill many important functions. Among these are:

THEY PRODUCE WATER-SOLUBLE SHORT-CHAIN FATTY ACIDS (with only 4–5 carbon atoms) like butyric acid and valeric acid, which are easily absorbed by and nourish the intestinal wall. This strengthens the intestinal wall's barrier function and stops fecal content (i.e., toxins, dead or living bacteria, or bacterial remains) from leaking into the body.

THEY EXTRACT LOTS OF WHOLESOME SUBSTANCES—antioxidants, vitamins, important amino acids, and energy—from, among other things, the fresh plant leaves we eat. Then these are sent into the body. Sugar is among these substances, which is also important for the body's and the brain's function. However, this sugar is slowly absorbed over several hours.

In conclusion, it can be said that Gram-positive and Gram-negative bacteria show totally different "social" behavioral patterns. When there is a lack of nourishment, and the environment is unsuitable, the Gram-positives bow out politely and disappear quietly.

This makes it easy for the gram-negatives to quickly take over, programming the immune system toward increased inflammation. They don't just stay in the intestine, but infiltrate the rest of the body with toxins, bacteria (living or dead), and bacterial remains. Eventually they will change the body's metabolism. So it is of utmost importance to quickly overturn this takeover. There is plenty to do in your life and body to make the Gram+ bacteria able to retake command and displace Gram– bacteria!

Apart from eating a diet rich in magnesium, you can provide Gram+ bacteria further assistance by using dietary supplements like probiotics that provide the gut with supplementary protective bacteria.

However, don't forget that probably 80 percent of the probiotics sold are totally useless. By examining many of the health claims related to different probiotic preparations, the EFSA (European Food Safety Authority) has shown most of the examined probiotic strains/species lack the health-promoting properties the producers/sellers promise.

Educate yourself and get objective information before you commit to a product!

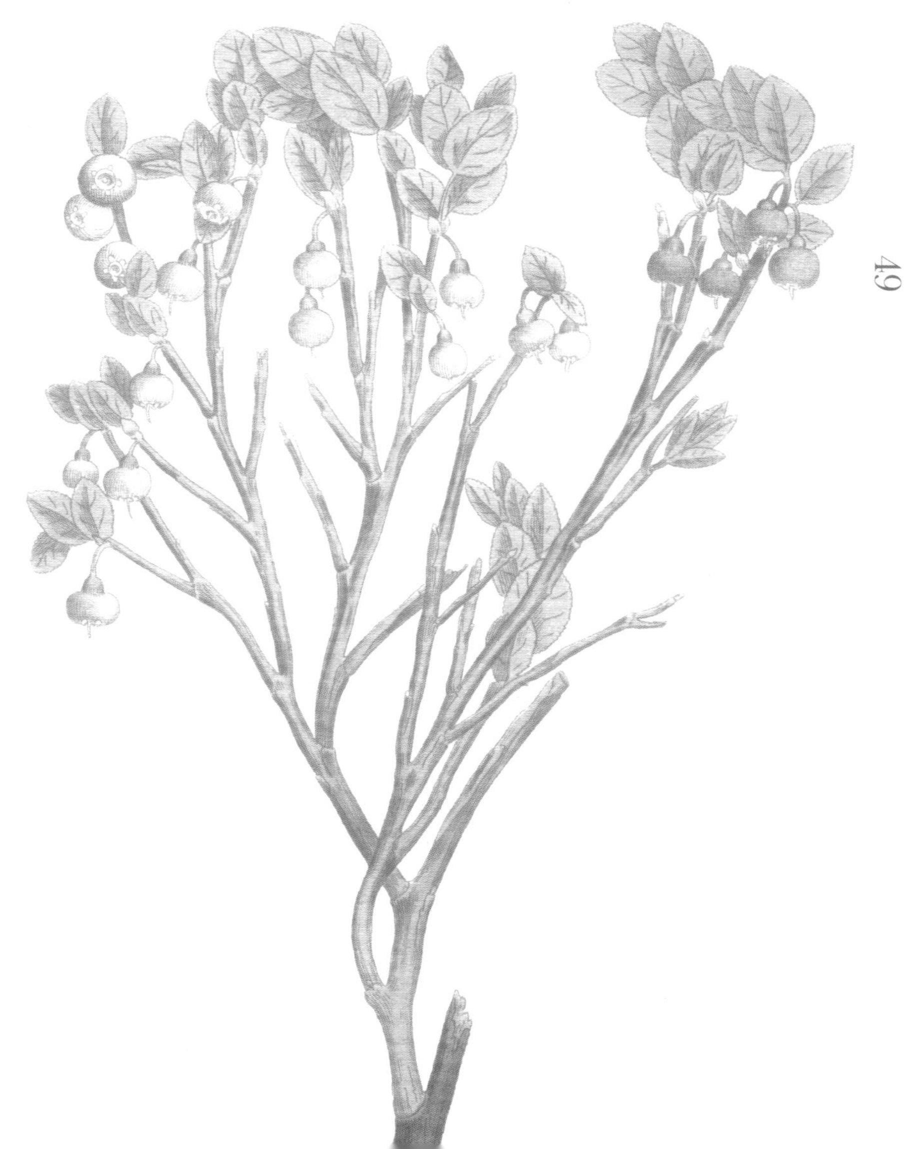

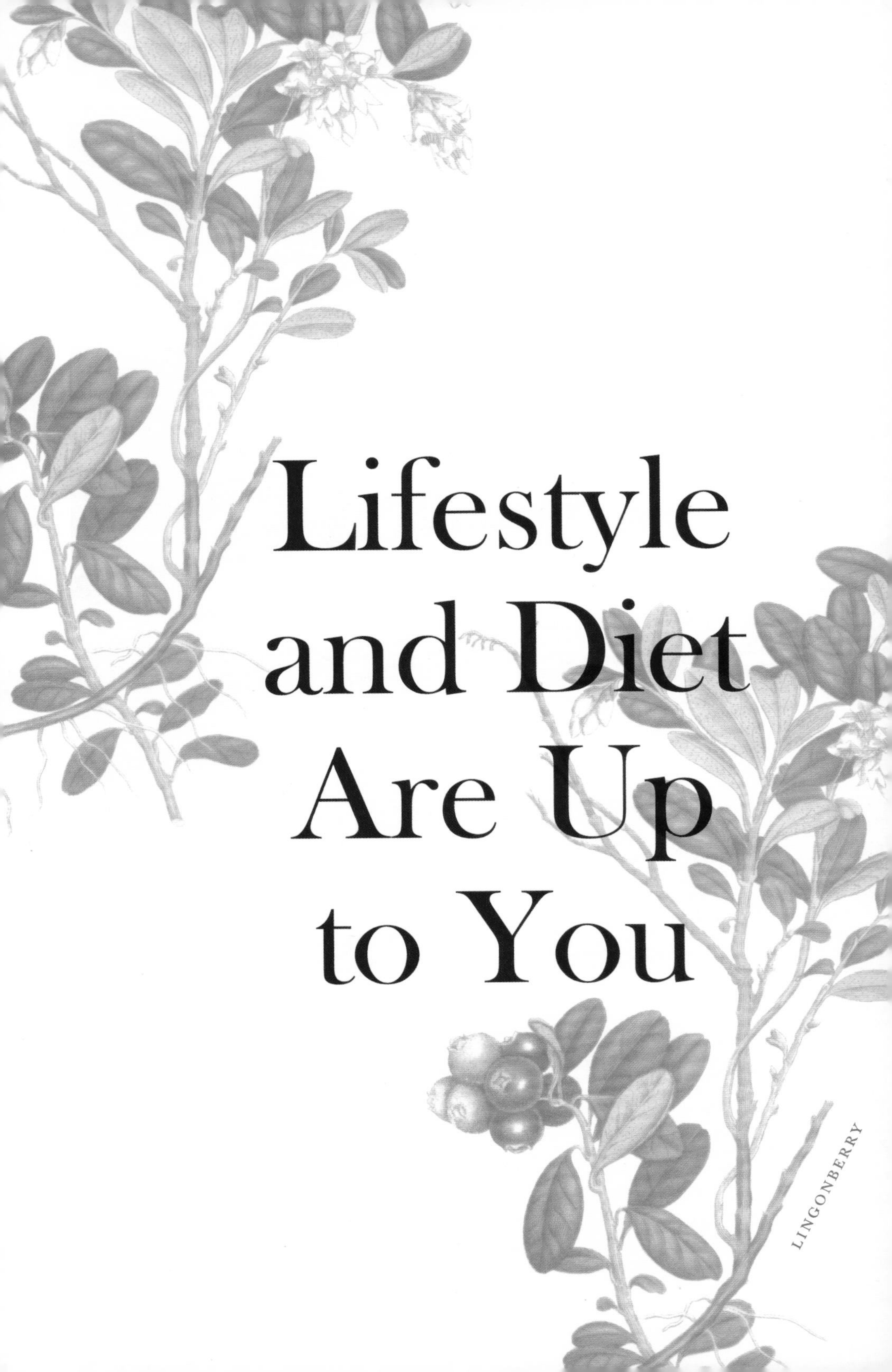

Lifestyle and Diet Are Up to You

03

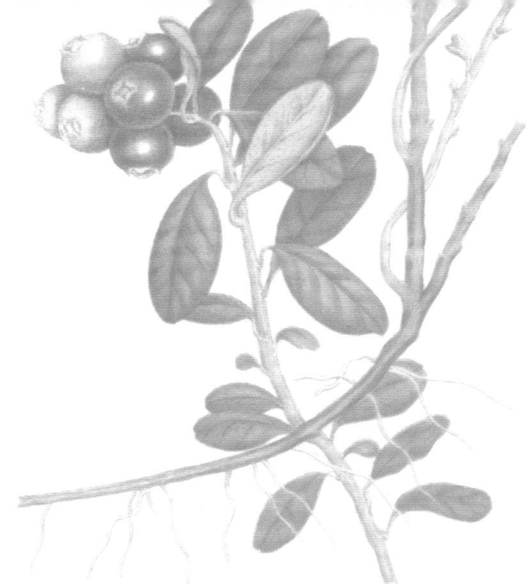

My thoughts about the correlation between the gut and health are receiving strong support from the international research community today. I also receive invaluable feedback from countless followers on my home page and on Facebook.

In this chapter, I'll give an overview of the Anti-Inflammatory Diet Solution's method, what it means, and what characterizes a gut-friendly diet.

Here's an important starting point: Contrary to what many believe, family history and genetics are not at all such deciding factors in health. Habits, however, play a big role.

So, if you want to get healthier: Change your dietary habits!

IT IS A widespread misunderstanding that biological inheritance and genetics play a big part in disease origins. We have had the same genes for hundreds of thousands, even millions of years. Many of today's commonly found diseases have been conspicuously absent for centuries. It's true there might be an inherited tendency for a specific illness—but it is often a provocative lifestyle that makes it poke up its head.

It is really habits, not family history, that put their stamp on people's health.

Studies performed with identical twins, primarily in Japan, have contributed vital information about the importance of lifestyle compared to genetics. (As you know, identical twins have identical genetic material.) Twins, where one twin had moved to the United States while the other stayed in Japan, were studied. The researchers discovered it was nearly always the twin who moved to a foreign country and changed their lifestyle who developed chronic illness.

The Force of Habit

Both the Old Testament and other writings from the time describe that illness often collects among certain individuals, families, groups, and peoples. We can observe big differences among groups and individuals even today.

Another observation that is less talked about: if a family member develops a chronic illness, other members of the same family, most often the spouse, run a greater risk of also developing a chronic illness.

It is also well documented that individuals of a lower socioeconomic class (low income and low educational level) run nearly double the risk of developing illness compared to individuals of a higher socioeconomic class (higher income, higher educational level). The increased rate of illness in the underprivileged class also affects children.

Most noticed, however, was the big difference in the amount of illness between countries. For instance, the United States has a significantly increased morbidity rate compared with Japan—it varied from approximately double the rate of cardiovascular disease to approximately three to four times the level for breast and prostate cancer.

All these observations strengthen our picture of how important lifestyle is for health. It can break it down or build it up, and how your lifestyle affects your health is very much up to you. Access to health-related information is important. Deciding to change your lifestyle for your health, therefore, benefits from your will to incorporate and apply the knowledge you find.

Reduce Overindulgence

Today we have a pretty good idea of what is good and what is bad for our health. The insights have been arrived at through, among other things, hundreds of thousands of animal experiments and epidemiological studies.

Here are some examples of foods that have a negative effect on your health if you eat too much of them.

CALORIES
SUGAR
SATURATED FATS
TRANS FATS
OMEGA-6
RED MEAT
DAIRY PRODUCTS

Perhaps the most important health-promoting action is not just avoiding overindulgence but also eating substantially less than you believe you really want. This means that all healthy individuals ought to try to eat a lot less than they do habitually. All healthy people need to reevaluate the motto "eat to satiety." For clarification, I'm of course not directing this at people suffering from eating disorders.

A clear example of the health benefits of calorie restraint: When the caloric intake for rats and mice was reduced to a third of what they wanted, they didn't just get healthier, their life span increased by 70 percent.

The same observations have been seen with apes. Few studies have been done on humans, but the ones that have been done point to essentially improved health conditions in the persons who had the stamina to practice this lifestyle for several years. Most of us, myself included, need to be very determined to be able to practice this knowledge over the long term.

Nearly a quarter million fats are known in the chemical world. Some of them—the animal saturated fats such as omega-6 (prolific in cheap industrial oils like sunflower oil) have, without a doubt, negative effects on health. On the other hand, others like omega-3 have shown proven positive effects.

Even if we have backed off lately from some warnings regarding the negative effects of saturated fat on cardiovascular health, high consumption of these fats is still strongly associated with, among other disorders, the occurrence of certain cancers.

The different toxins and hormones that accompany the food and that are often stored in our body's adipose tissue increase the negative influence of animal fats.

Scientists and health authorities agree that trans fats, created when vegetable oils are heated to high temperatures and used, for instance, in industrial margarine production and industrial baking, have strongly negative effects on health. Trans fats are currently, or are in the process of being, prohibited in many countries.

Large intake of red meat also demonstrates strong negative effects, especially when the meat is from animals fed concentrated feed. Some studies show this with meat ingestion more than twice weekly. Especially negative was the consumption of cured meats (i.e., meatballs, hamburgers, sausage, and bacon).

We'll return to the negative effects of the Western diet, but I want to focus on health-bringing messages (i.e., what we ourselves, with simple means, can do to change things for the better). In this, it is all about three important things:

- More about how vegetables, *plants*, have shown themselves since immemorial times to be healthy for humans
- More about how raw vegetables are the least destroyed food we can find
- More about how the heating of food should be used as little as possible

Outsmart Sugar

Sugar is insidious. Lots of manufactured foods are made sweeter. Outsmart the sugar! Check the sugar content in the ingredients list.

Sugar consumed in a restrained amount is an important energy source. However, an excess of sugar, or sugar-like foods, creates serious health problems. Refined industrial sugar is nearly exclusively absorbed only in the small intestine.

"An excess of sugar or sugar-like foods creates serious health problems."

Two lists from the Consumer Association in Stockholm show the high levels of sugar in common foods. Avoid these foods if you want the best for your children and yourself. (Some dairy products contain more sugar than the 1 ounce (25 g) per ½ cup (100 ml) that is the daily intake for adults as recommended by the WHO [World Health Organization]). Serve instead a homemade muesli with some fruit. Try Bircher muesli, which we like a lot. However, we don't eat it until lunchtime, giving our stomachs a rest from any form of calories during the morning hours.

Some commercial probiotic drinks also contain far too much sugar. Avoid them!

Minimize sugar in the diet, especially fructose and sugar-like foods: marmalades, jam, bread, cookies and cakes, pizza, pasta, refined rice, even warm potatoes and warm root vegetables. You can eat more potatoes and root vegetables if you let them cool down first (because the sugar reverts to fiber).

FROM MY TWELVE COMMANDMENTS FOR OPTIMAL HEALTH, P. 74

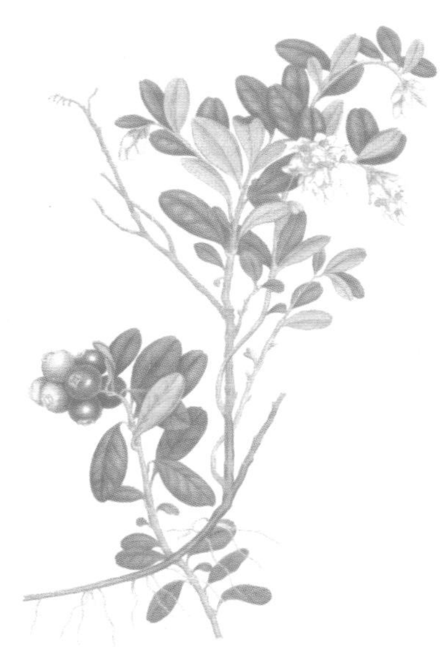

Also be careful with fruit juices as well as ripe yellow bananas—these are nearly pure sugar. However, a green banana is full of fiber. It is at its best when you can hardly peel it. In Asia they eat yellow bananas to put on weight and green bananas when they want to lose weight, and it seems to work!

Turn up your nose at coffee klatches with sweet buns and cakes, and don't frequent pastry shops—if you haven't already stopped.

In my opinion, these ancient habits of coffee meet-ups with cakes and cookies are a part of the past and should have their place in a museum. It is more wholesome to offer your friends a glass of wine—preferably red wine as it is rich in antioxidants and very low in sugar.

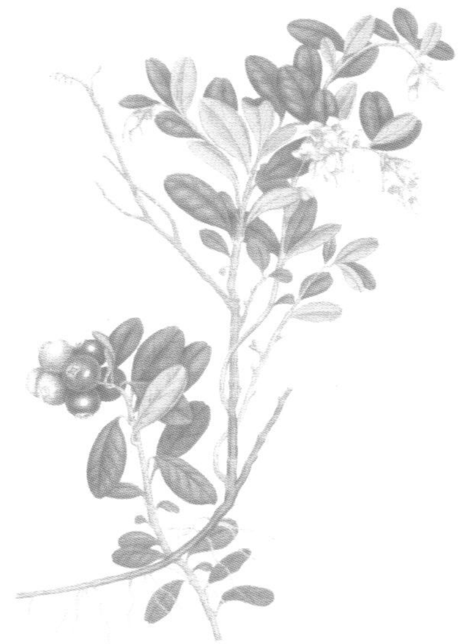

Early Wisdom—and Today's Decay

Before we had today's modern healthcare, the sick were treated and looked after by the church and the cloisters. Health was looked for in plants and plant ingredients from the big monastery gardens—similar to what was already practiced during antiquity. It is impressive to read books written by Hildegard von Bingen, a nun who led a few cloisters in twelfth-century Germany. In the books she describes in detail the healing characteristics of different plants and gives recipes for using them for food. The book *Physica* is all about health and healing and describes in depth how they experienced the healing properties of different plants. This really isn't that different from today's perception.

Even long after the construction of modern hospitals and the advent of pharmaceuticals, the selection in the pharmacies mainly originated in the plant kingdom.

Unfortunately, scientists in the twentieth century were drawn to search for more sweetness in foods. They started refining traditional fruits so as to make them taste sweeter. This happened in a time before we were made aware of sugar's detrimental effect on health. In hindsight, we can wish this had never happened. To reverse this path seems impossible, and that applies to the refinement of all other edible plants we use for food. Instead, we have to ration our consumption of fruits we traditionally ate lots of. The suggestion is to eat at most half an ounce (15 g) of fructose a day—the equivalent of not more than three apples, pears, or oranges.

There is also an intensive search for grains that have better nutritional value than commonly found in overprocessed grains. The same ambitions also concern our fruits. Some new fruits with great health characteristics have lately found their way to our tables.

I'll return later with effusive praise for the avocado!

Raw Food Is Best

Food is very sensitive to manipulation and easily loses a lot of its nutrition. Thirty minutes after a head of lettuce has been cut from its roots, half of its antioxidants have disappeared. That is one of the reasons why many plants in the produce section are sold with their roots still attached.

For thousands of years the earth's population has used plants to keep and restore health. Plants, just like bacteria, have existed on earth much longer than humans. The ones that survived eradication developed an immune system that is better, at least in some respects, than what humans possess. Such plants constitute a necessary complement for the human immune system and its defense against disease. It would be difficult to imagine human life without access to plants and bacteria.

Plants, with their rich content of immune-regulating fiber and antioxidants, as well as benign bacteria, rule the human immune system. In nature there exist about 200,000 different kinds of plants and a large number of different kinds of benign bacteria. However, there are less than five hundred plants regularly used as food, and only about a few dozen bacteria that have shown to have health-enhancing properties.

Knowing this, it becomes important to strive for the widest possible diversity of plant matter in our diet.

"Most fruits and vegetables can and ought to be eaten raw."

Heat treatment also quickly destroys many temperature sensitive ingredients in our food. Studies have shown that microwaving destroys approximately 97 percent of all antioxidants in fruit and vegetables. Olive oil, as an example, must not be heated above 82.4°F (28°C), to ensure it retains valuable wholesomeness. A lot of enzymes in food disappear at 104°F (40°C).

Many new synthetic substances start to form at 176°F (80°C), a process that is accelerated the more heat is increased with food preparation.

At high temperatures—like those needed for the pasteurization of milk or baking and toasting bread—considerable amounts of toxic substances are created that over time can have very negative effects on health.

This knowledge has brought on a change in many people's food preparation. Many avoid frying and grilling food. Instead, they prepare food—especially meat and fish—in a slow oven (i.e., at a low temperature and over several hours) or by careful steaming.

Fruit and vegetables should be heated as little as possible. After all, most fruits and vegetables can and ought to be eaten raw.

Don't Smoke with Your Stomach!

During school's chemistry lessons, pupils learn that heating leads to the creation of synthetic processes. These processes make it possible for new substances to form by "marrying" two or more substances—an opportunity that today's food industry and all households practice frequently. When ingredients are exposed to temperatures above 176°F to 212°F (80–100°C) they acquire totally new properties than the original and become toxic, even if only mildly.

According to the American Lung Association, more than four thousand new chemicals are generated when tobacco is heated.

The same thing happens, in principle, to our food when we heat it. If it were not so rich in nicotine, the tobacco plant would be one of our most wholesome plants. However, in the end, it is not the nicotine that is the main reason why tobacco use causes increased frequency of different diseases! It's the industrial manufacturing of tobacco—which comprises heating—that bears the biggest responsibility. In the manufacturing of tobacco more than a hundred substances are added. When heated, these substances join and create new substances which are noxious for health. These accumulate in the body, and they are difficult to expel from the body even if you stop smoking.

That explains why, decades later, former smokers still run a higher risk of being affected with different chronic illnesses than those who have never smoked.

The French scientist Louis Camille Maillard suggested in the 1900s that heating food led to the creation of new substances, and he likened them to what forms when smoking tobacco. He also proposed that the body's accumulation of these might be the cause of many chronic illnesses, especially kidney disease. His work was recognized and he received the French Academy of Medicine Award. However, everything was done to quickly suppress the new knowledge he presented.

It was during the last twenty years that interest in these substances has dramatically increased. We must thank the young scientific field of molecular biology for this. Through its methods we can investigate the substances' action mechanisms in the human body.

The substances in question are a kind of soot/carbon. It has been known for centuries that soot will not leave the body. These substances are usually black, gray, or brown. Foods with these shades of color are often rich in illness-provoking substances. There also exist white soot substances in dairy products that are found primarily in milk powder. AGE—short for advanced glycation end products—is a chemical reaction between carbohydrates and protein, while ALE—advanced lipooxidation end products—is the synthesis between carbohydrates and fats/lipids.

These substances gather, in theory, throughout the body, but mainly in certain internal organs. Something they all have in common is that they are self-radiating. The human eye cannot perceive this but it is fully possible to measure with a special instrument. Elevated content of these end products in the body is associated with illnesses—everything from Alzheimer's disease to various eye diseases in the elderly.

Collect Antioxidants

We already know that antioxidants in fruit and vegetables possess the characteristic to counteract the otherwise harmful oxidation from so-called free radicals.

However, fire (heat) doesn't just destroy the good bacteria in food but also food's antioxidants. That's why daily consumption of a large amount of raw and fresh plant matter is so critical. In many countries the government urges the population to eat up to eight fresh fruits and vegetables daily, of which at least half should be vegetables.

Certain plants contain a great amount of antioxidants—but can only be ingested in small amounts (spices, for instance). Plants with fewer antioxidants, therefore, are more important, because they can easily be consumed in servings of 3½ ounces (100 g) or more.

The next page shows you a selection of antioxidant-rich foods. The numbers show the amount of antioxidants as measured by ORAC (oxygen radical absorbance capacity) per 3½ oz (100 g).

Frequent use of spices, preferably fresh, is important. It is also wise to regularly eat fresh berries and vegetables such as broccoli, spinach, kale, and onion—as well as nuts, beans, lentils, and peas. All these foods provide substantial supplements of both natural antioxidants and fiber.

Lately, berries like acai, maqui, and goji have received lots of attention due to their high levels of antioxidants. However, there is no evidence that they are inherently better for health compared with freshly picked berries that can be found in our forests and nature. Sometimes our berries can also be bought more cheaply than the exotic berries, and they don't have to be transported long distances from foreign parts of the world.

"The potato is wholesome when it is eaten cold or cooled down."

GO AHEAD AND USE THESE ANTIOXIDANT-RICH INGREDIENTS

ORAC µmol TE/3 1/2 OZ (100 G)

DRIED SPICES—clove 315,000, oregano 201,000, turmeric 160,000, cumin 77,000, parsley 74,000, curry 48,500, mustard seeds and ginger 29,000, black peppercorn 27,600

FRESH SPICES—staghorn sumac 86,800, sage 32,000, thyme 27,400, dill 4,400

BEVERAGES—cacao powder 81,000, yerba tea 5,000, red wine 4,800, green tea 1,200 to 2,000, black tea 700 to 1,200, rooibos tea 800, decaffeinated tea 700 to 800

FRUITS—prunes 8,050, dried raisins 2,800, dried figs 3,200, apples 4,280, oranges 2,100, white grapefruit 1,240, cherries 3,750, kiwi 860, red grapefruit 1,640

BERRIES—acai 102,500, maqui 19,900, goji 25,000, sea buckthorn 22,500, elder 14,500, plums 8,050, bilberries 9,600, raspberries 5,000, strawberries 4,300, red/white/black currants 3,400

NUTS—pecans 17,900, walnuts 13,500, hazelnuts (filberts) 9,600

VEGETABLES—kale 1,770, spinach 1,500, red onion and garlic 1,520, Brussels sprouts 2,000, alfalfa 1,930, broccoli 3,080, red beets 1,850, yellow onion 1,450, red bell pepper 935, eggplant 400

FIBER-RICH SEEDS—staghorn sumac 312,400, tannin durrah 45,400 to 240,000, rice fiber 24,300, flaxseed 19,600

Instead of using expensive imported berries, it is a good idea to eat local berries and vegetables, of course, daily. Remember also to choose your vegetables according to the season. They are both better tasting and cheaper that way.

Certain antioxidants like lycopene in tomatoes require some heating to be released. Some antioxidants, like glutathione, survive heating, even if they are very much reduced. Glutathione is often called the master antioxidant and is in rich supply in broccoli and potatoes.

Root vegetables are especially important because of their rich fiber content. Daily consumption of root vegetables, such as different kinds of cabbage and onion, is highly recommended.

It is important to remember that the wholesome potato—which many avoid due to its higher calorie content—is especially healthy when it is consumed cold or cooled down. When the potato is allowed to cool down, its sugar recrystallizes and slow-acting carbohydrate resistance starch is created. The same process is at work in several other root vegetables and broccoli.

Reduce or eliminate heat-induced inflammation-provoking proteins/heat-generated toxins (i.e., glycated and lipid-oxidation end products). Never heat food to more than 248°F to 266°F (120°C–130°C).

FROM MY TWELVE COMMANDS FOR OPTIMAL HEALTH. P. 74

Omega-3? Well, of Course!

Omega-3 is an important dietary supplement, usually taken in capsule form. Got questions? For the doubter, or someone who isn't read up on the subject, here is how you can explain the vital intake of omega-3:

The human body is incredibly clever at producing most of the substances it needs, but it is unable to make certain necessities, among them the fatty acid omega-3. These substances have to come through the diet and are called *essential*—vital. There are essential amino acids and essential fatty acids.

The essential amino acids are the building blocks we need to be able to create certain proteins. There are eight amino acids for adults and ten for children. It only takes one missing amino acid for the production of the desired protein to stop immediately. One of these essential amino acids is tryptophan, which is crucial for synthesis of the important neurotransmitters serotonin and melatonin—important for wakefulness, sleep, energy, and physical activity.

The essential fatty acids CLA (conjugated linoleic acid) and linoleic acid are vital for building cell walls and for regulating levels of inflammation in the body.

THE BIG FAT CHAOS

For many hundreds of thousands of years humanity had a diet that contained just over 20 percent fat. I believe we can posit that humans are genetically suited for such a diet. During the last 150 to 200 years they have, however, dramatically increased the consumption of dairy products and different meats. This has brought with it a near doubling of fat consumption—see the picture on the next page! This development has contributed significantly to the increased level of chronic inflammation in our bodies.

Today there are groups of people the world over who have chosen to massively increase the fat content in their diet. The method is called LCHF. The letters stand for low carb/high fat, which means a low intake of carbohydrates and high intake of fat. A low consumption of carbohydrate is extremely beneficial if it is limited to "refined" carbohydrates: sugar and sugar-like foods like bread

MORE FAT, LESS NUTRIENTS

People's fat consumption has increased enormously through history, while at the same time the consumption of what is wholesome has declined. Below is our fat consumption in comparison with consumption of vitamin C and E since prehistoric times.

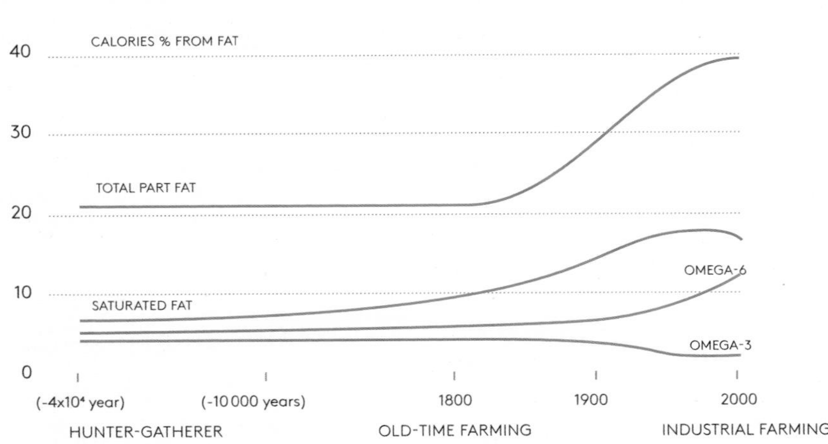

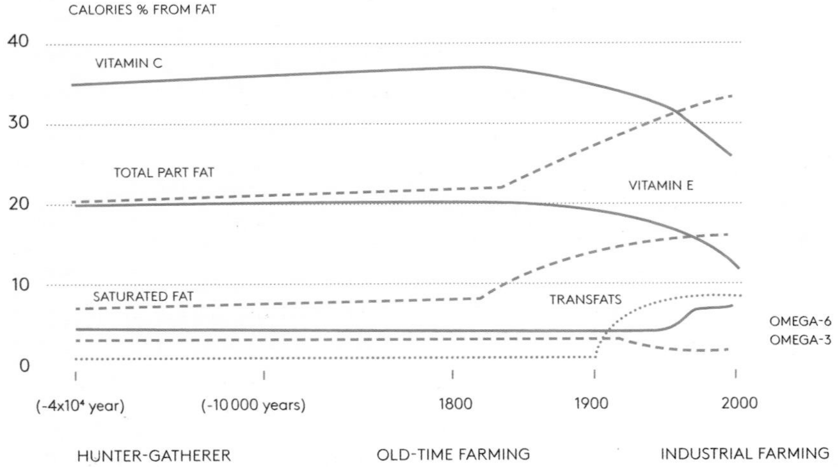

(both white and dark), cooked warm root vegetables, rice, pasta, pizza, candy, and sodas. LCHF is also an excellent weight-loss method. But the large intake of fat will undoubtedly be catastrophic for health in the long term.

I would have preferred to see the method called RCRF, that is, right carbohydrates (green and unprocessed) and right fats (short-chain and medium-chain fatty acids)—the ones that are taken up via the portal vein and don't have to pass through the thoracic duct and cause postprandial inflammation.

> "I would have preferred that the LCHF method was called RCRF, that is, right carbohydrates (green and unprocessed) and right fats."

In the last 150 to 200 years we have doubled our intake of saturated long-chain fat, increased our consumption of dairy products approximately 5,000 percent, and taken our sugar consumption from less than a pound (500 g) a year (1850) to nearly 88 pounds (40 kg) a year. This is an increase of nearly 10,000 percent. Simultaneously, the intake of toxic trans fats, acrylamide toxins, and environmental toxins, has dramatically increased in many countries.

Our consumption of cheap seed oils, primarily sunflower oil, has brought a manyfold increase of Omega-6 fats, which are just as necessary as omega-3 fats. However, the former have an "inflammation" demarcation boundary—at the same time as our consumption of omega-3 fats (active anti-inflammation) is halved. At the moment this balance is heavily unbalanced in favor of inflammation. In Sweden the ratio is somewhere along 1:3 or 1:4. In the United States, which is further along the slippery slope to ill health, it is around 1:10 or worse.

PRACTICAL DIETARY SUPPLEMENTS

Admittedly, there are studies that question the importance of balance between omega-3 and omega-6, which complicates the recommendations often given. For me personally, the use of omega-3 is self-evident.

Here's new evidence: An animal study published in 2017—unfortunately only in Chinese—shows a significantly improved gut flora and reduced level of endotoxins in the blood with regular supplementation with omega-3. In great probability, this means a substantial reduction in postprandial inflammation after meals.

A daily dose of three grams (1⁄10 oz) of omega-3 has so far been the norm for users. Omega-6 is more than likely supplied to the brim through the diet and it seldom needs to be supplemented. In fact, it's advisable to use certain restraint with omega-6, especially regarding sunflower oil.

We never use refined oils in our family—not even olive oil. Our small consumption of oil is only of medium-chain fatty acids, MCT oils, mostly coconut oil. Even though sunflower oil and olive oil are long-chain and are forced to go through the thoracic duct, they are not considered as aggressive for the blood vessel interior as the animal fats.

Natural omega-3 is found primarily in fatty fish such as salmon, mackerel, sill, and sardines; certain algae; and, for example, walnuts.

It is easy to get a daily 1⁄10-ounce (3 g) dose of omega-3 by either taking 1⁄6 ounce (5 g) fish oil, 1⁄3 ounce (10 g) flaxseed oil, 3½ ounces (100 g) salmon, 1¾ ounces (50 g) walnuts, or 2 ounces (60 g) mackerel—but it is much more difficult to get a sufficient amount from other foods. For example, you would need to eat 2¼ pounds (1 kg) of almonds, shrimp, or white fish, 14¼ pounds (6½ kg) of cucumber, or 17½ pounds of apples to cover your daily need for omega-3.

I find it more practical to take omega-3 as a dietary supplement.

KRILL, A HIGHLY INTERESTING OIL

Lately there's been an increased interest in using krill oil as a source for omega-3. Krill are a shrimp-like whale food, of which about 500 million metric tons are caught in the North Atlantic each year. Krill oil is extra rich in the omega-3 fats EPA (eicosapentaenoic acid) and DHA (docosahexaenoic acid). While both EPA and DHA occur in common fish oil in the form of triglycerides, it is the phospholipid structure in krill oil that is seen as a considerable advantage.

Krill oil also contains relatively large amounts of vitamin E, vitamin A, vitamin D, and the pigment canthaxanthin, which gives krill oil a forty-eight times stronger antioxidant effect than fish oil. Krill oil fills an important place in the fight against general inflammation. Regular consumption of omega-3, and especially krill oil, may noticeably reduce:

- high level of blood fats—and blood glucose to a degree
- oxidative stress, high levels of inflammation in the body, and also high level of CRP (C-reactive protein), an indicator of a wide-ranging high level of inflammation in the body
- hunger, obesity, and metabolic syndrome/diabetes
- chronic kidney disease
- skeletal and joint pain, especially rheumatoid arthritis (RA)
- menstrual pain and premenstrual pain (premenstrual syndrome—PMS)
- cancer pain and emaciation due to cancer (certain observations also report reduced cancer progression)
- memory loss, aging of the brain, and ADHD (attention deficit hyperactivity disorder)

I'll return to the metabolic syndrome phenomena several times later on.

Treat Yourself to Vitamin D!

It has long been known that the frequency of infections and chronic illness increases the nearer to the North or South Pole you live. Recently published studies show that Africans who live in rural villages have a much higher level of vitamin D than what we see in Northern Europe.

We have also long been astonished that persons with dark skin who move to more northern latitudes, especially to North America and Northern Europe, are considerably more often struck by illness than lighter-skinned persons.

Lately these observations have gotten their elucidation when it has been shown that these individuals often suffer from a lack of vitamin D. The amount of vitamin D we get from our diet (primarily from fatty fish and canola oil) is miniscule compared to what we receive from the sun.

Most people along high latitudes don't get sufficient amounts of vitamin D from the sun during the winter months, the darkest months of the year. At the same time the body's deposit of vitamin D is being halved every six weeks. High doses of sunlight at the same time mean an increased risk of skin cancer. Northern inhabitants, especially those with underlying illness causing sensitivity to sunshine, should opt for vitamin D as a *dietary supplement*—rather than burn through unlimited sun exposure.

The body's access to vitamin D is at its lowest when daylight hours are the shortest. This might explain why many illnesses like depression and intestinal inflammations readily start or reoccur during the winter in the US. Clinical studies suggest that a normally elevated level of vitamin D brings a radically reduced frequency of infections; for instance, during surgical interventions and also improved survival rate after cancer surgeries. In addition, vitamin D prevents a lowering of cognitive function, incidences of depression, and mortality from cardiovascular disease or brain hemorrhage.

CONTROLS HUNDREDS OF PROCESSES

The history of vitamin D deficiency is long and filled with indescribable torments. In the middle of the eighteenth century this insufficiency was called *rachitis* (rickets) worldwide, and in Sweden we called it the English disease. The lack of vitamin D made the skeleton soft. If this was not treated, the bones would stay deformed for life.

We know nowadays that vitamin D isn't just a vitamin, it is also a powerful hormone, and, above all else a deciding factor for a well-functioning microbiome and its immune functions. It is just lately that these properties have gotten their proper recognition. The effectiveness is amplified when a generous amount of vitamin K2 is present—it is a true healing vitamin.

The main interest for a long time has been vitamin D's capacity to aid the storage of minerals such as calcium and magnesium in the skeleton. Only a small addition of vitamin D was apparently needed for these functions. That explains why a low daily dose was long recommended for children and adults. However, to maintain a well-functioning microbiome, and an optimally functioning immune system, it seems like considerably higher levels are needed!

A mild vitamin D deficiency seems to be the rule rather than the exception in Sweden. It has been reported that more than 80 percent of children and adolescents in upper Norrland [the north of Sweden] and more than 60 percent in the south of Sweden have confirmed vitamin D deficiency.

It is organs like parathyroid, brain, kidneys, intestine, microbiome, and skeleton that are particularly sensitive to low levels of vitamin D. Main sources of dietary vitamin D are fatty fish, eggs, and whole milk—but nobody can consume the large amounts of fatty fish or eggs that would be needed.

One hour full-body exposure/sunbathing in the middle of the day gives approximately 24,000 IE of vitamin D. (IE is the international unit where 1 µg vitamin D is the equivalent of 40 IE). It is partly a misunderstanding that you shouldn't sunbathe at midday. Quite the opposite, you should—but carefully and without burning! The sun has two different kinds of rays, the harmful carcinogenic UV-1 and the healthy UV-2. The ratio between healthy/harmful UV rays is at its absolute best in the middle of the day. It is better, therefore, to sunbathe for a short time at midday than for a longer time earlier or later in the day. You do get some more harmful rays but absorb immensely more of the healthy rays!

VITAMIN D DEFICIENCY IS A HIGHWAY TO DISEASE

Studies show that the majority of individuals who arrive at the hospital suffering from a chronic illness also suffer from a vitamin D deficiency: pre-bariatric surgery for obesity 57 percent (fair-skinned) and 79 percent (dark-skinned), and pre-kidney transplantation 67 percent (fair-skinned) and 95 percent (dark-skinned).

How interesting it would be to know how many of these treatments could have been avoided if a vitamin D deficiency had been treated earlier in the patient's life.

Vitamin D has a phenomenal ability to hold off influenza, which so regularly affects people in the spring when the body's vitamin D levels are at their lowest. There is no medicine that can compete with vitamin D at staving this off.

An American-European research project (using methods produced by Health of Economics Professor Bengt Jönsson at Stockholm School of Economics [SSE] in Stockholm, Sweden) examined what effect it would have if everybody within the European Union had sufficient levels of vitamin D in their blood.

It turned out it would result in a likely reduction of illness. One estimate was cardiovascular disease (mostly heart attacks and stroke) would decrease up to 14 percent, infections including influenza up to 7 percent, type 2 diabetes up to 7 percent, cancer 6.4 percent, osteoporosis approximately 1.5 percent, and multiple sclerosis at least 1 percent.

Did these new findings create excited activity among Europe's health politicians? Alas, not at all.

THE CORRECT LEVEL OF VITAMIN D?

A supplement of 400 IE of vitamin D was once needed to eradicate rachitis. Today many researchers feel that a daily dose of ten times as much—2,000 to 4,000 IE—could result in great opportunities to reduce obesity, infections, and chronic illness.

The EFSA Scientific Committee for the European Union recommends a standard daily consumption of up to 2,000 IE daily for adults and 1,000 IE for children.

The big problem with this is that there exists considerable individual differences. For instance, I have followed athletes who carefully monitor their vitamin D levels. Even though they ingest large amounts, they still find it very difficult to reach the desired levels.

The intake is improved if you simultaneously consume fat, but it doesn't solve the problem completely. Researchers agree that older individuals with thinner epidermis possess an inferior ability to create vitamin D and inferior uptake so they need a larger dose—most probably double. My wife Marianne's uptake of vitamin D is, for example, better than mine. Her values are really at the levels of someone who lives by the equator, while mine are a quarter less. We take 3,000 to 5,000 IE daily the year round.

Imagine if health clinics could test for vitamin D levels in a simpler way and more frequently? I often argue the importance of practicing proactive healthcare to prevent expensive disease care. I can only continue to nag on the subject and hope that our politicians will one day realize the savings that can be had.

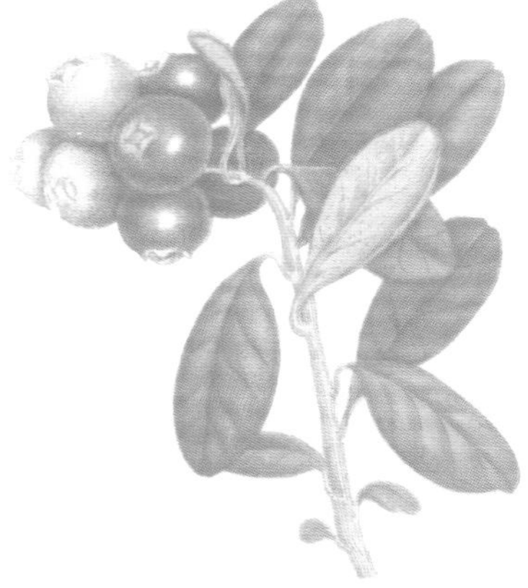

My Twelve Commandments for Optimal Health

HERE I'VE COLLECTED and developed the best advice I can share with a fellow human being.

These are twelve commandments for those of you who want to boost your intestinal health and stay healthy.

The optimal health has to be supported sturdily by three legs: Daily exercise, proper diet, and stress control. As I'm directing my research to the intestines and not toward exercise or stress, the focus of my commandments is care of your microbiome.

Nevertheless, I'm absolutely convinced that collaboration of all three legs is essential. The inferior Western diet we together are going to fight is intimately associated with sedentary living and stress.

I'll do my best and you'll do yours!

1 Minimize sugar in the diet, especially fructose; also sugar-like foods: marmalade, jam, bread, cookies and cakes, pizza, pasta, polished rice, even warm potatoes and warm root vegetables. If you let the root vegetables and potatoes cool down before you eat them, you can eat more of them (the sugar turns into resistant starch).

2 Reduce or eliminate all dairy products—especially butter, cheese, and powdered milk.

3 Limit the consumption of meat to, at most, 3/4 pound (300 g) a week. Avoid processed meat: smoked, fried, grilled, sausage, meatballs, hamburgers, and similar items. Also avoid meat from animals reared on concentrates. Look for grass-fed meat. Avoid farmed fish and look for wild-caught fish.

4 Limit or eliminate the consumption of long-chain fats: pork fat, beef fat (tallow), and oils like olive oil, canola oil, and sunflower oil. Replace them with medium-chain fats such as coconut oil and avocado oil.

5 Eliminate foods containing inflammation-provoking proteins: casein (dairy products), gluten (wheat, rye and barley), and zein (corn).

6 Reduce or eliminate heat-induced, inflammation-provoking proteins/heat toxins (glycated and lipid oxidated products). Never heat food above 248°F to 266°F.

7 Minimize contact with bacterial toxins such as endotoxins as well as different environmental toxins.

8 Reduce consumption of salt, both sodium and chloride. Increase intake of iodine, use iodized salt, and especially avoid fluor and bromine. Minimize contact with plastics and never heat plastic or plastic-covered items.

9 Minimize contact with chemicals. Avoid all nonessential pharmaceuticals and only use drugs for internal or external use when they are absolutely necessary.

10 Eat lots of plant foods—at least $1\frac{3}{4}$ pounds to $2\frac{1}{4}$ pounds a day. Eat the foods as fresh and raw as possible. Defrosted frozen foods are also good. Look for foods that are particularly rich in antioxidants, plant fiber, and plant protein. Use gluten-free grains like amaranth, durrah (sorghum), teff, quinoa, seeds, peas, beans, lentils, almonds, and nuts. Soak dried foods in water for 12 to 24 hours before eating them.

11 Aim to consume fresh or freshly frozen fruit and vegetables, and choose items with low glycemic index. Use lots of inflammation-inhibitory teas like pu-erh and yerba maté and inflammation-reducing spices: ground cloves, turmeric, and different kinds of peppers. Like chili pepper? Go for it! Eat whole olives, but avoid the oil. Supplement year-round with vitamin D, omega-3, turmeric, and probiotics/synbiotics—the four cornerstones of an anti-inflammatory regime. Go ahead and add sources of iodine such as potassium chloride or kelp.

12 Practice daily intermittent fasting, that is, restrict your eating window to approximately six hours out of the day through practicing what is sometimes called *skipping breakfast* (no calories before lunch) or *skipping dinner* (no calories after 2 p.m.).

How Principled Do You Have to Be?

Many people ask me how principled you have to be in following my commandments to succeed? My answer: Everybody who knows me knows that I follow my own commandments as closely as I can—and with great pleasure. Every day I am healthy reinforces my belief that my lifestyle is health promoting. I also have the advantage of sharing the interest in a gut-friendly diet with Marianne, who is a real ombudsperson for the gut microbiome. She watches carefully so there are no deviations. Why would you strive for less?

Nevertheless, dear reader, I know that everybody is different and has other possibilities than I do for following this lifestyle. Stay as principled as you can! Every step following the commandments is a step in the right direction. The most important thing here is to not forget to concentrate on raw plant foods, daily exercise, and guarding against mental stress.

If you can't carry out a radical change in your life and kitchen at this moment, focus on what is most important. Cut down on sugar consumption considerably, as well as dairy products and bad fats. Preferably avoid gluten. Remember omega-3, vitamin D, and iodine. Stick to the idea of daily exercise, even if it is only a walk in the neighborhood. Relish precious moments of peace when they appear (perhaps a rest from computer monitor and cell phone now and then).

Even I will compromise when I'm away from home if it becomes awkward or impolite to be too fussy.

Until a few years ago it was certainly much easier to follow all my own commandments. I wasn't especially social. All my time was spent in research, and I communicated mostly with scientific colleagues. But I have become a bit of a celebrity since the authors of *Food Pharmacy* hauled me out into the limelight. Now I have to weigh the principled role model demand against the need to be polite and available.

Perhaps you, dear reader, encounter similar situations with demands in between home and public life. If that's the case, I will happily share a few tips with you on how I navigate.

For example, I know that all eyes will be on me if I'm invited to a Christmas buffet. "Well, what's the gut professor going to choose from the dishes on the table?" Then I'll do like everybody else, I make a rough check: I search for foods that best fit my diet, but make a few small exceptions to not come over as too fussy.

I was recently invited to dinner at a well-known gourmet restaurant as a thank-you for a lecture. The host knew my diet profile and asked concernedly, "What can they get you, Stig?" I made a quick calculation: I realized that the restaurant was too good to work with processed foods, and I do eat both fish and some meat. I answered what seemed most convenient for all. "Thank you, I'll eat what they serve, but preferably without any gluten or dairy products."

We even make small compromises in our own kitchen. The small yolk in the mayonnaise, for example, is from a free-range hen, but it's still an animal source. If we want to use mayonnaise it will be good enough that we choose a good fat, coconut oil, and season it our own healthy way.

What is important is to not let the exception become the rule.

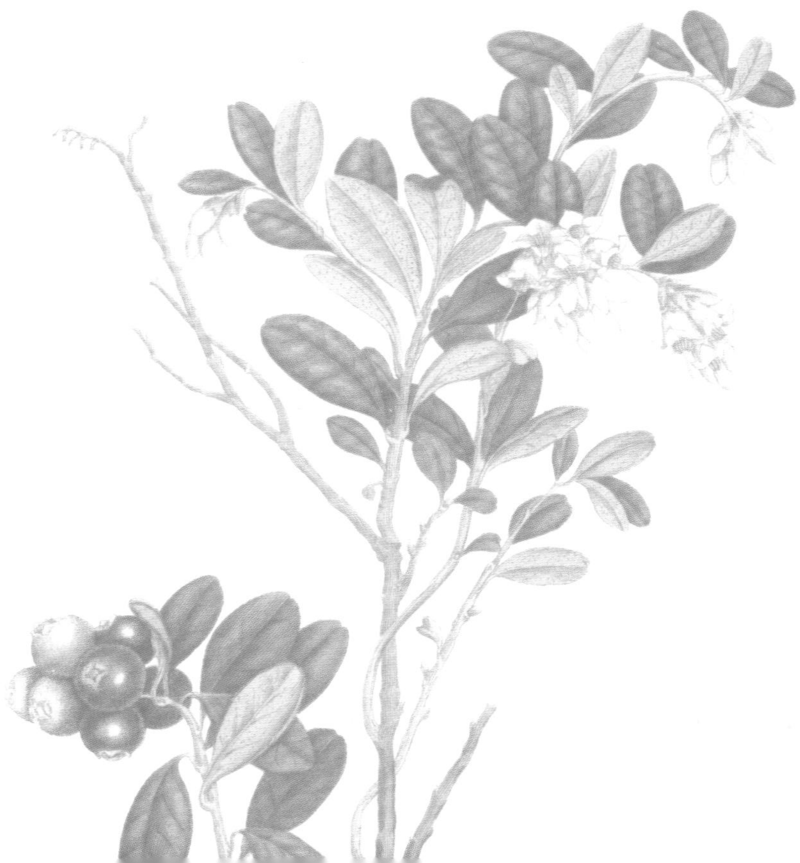

Three Basic Pillars: Exercise, Proper Diet, Stress Reduction

ARUGULA

04

We have so far talked a lot about the microbiome, and I'm sure you understand why. I am absolutely convinced that many more people would live a healthier and longer life if they knew more about how diet affects the digestive system and health.

Yet, my health method has a much wider focus than that. Your whole body must be engaged so you can eat yourself healthy! Your soul belongs here, too. Let me present the three pillars of the Anti-Inflammatory Diet Solution's method:

Plenty of exercise. Proper diet. Stress reduction.

IN A RUNNING COMPETITION consisting of long-distance runners with raw-food and non-raw-food diets, results were evident and not surprising. The winners were the ones who *both* ran and consumed plenty of raw plant foods. Without their raw-food diets, these runners might only have reached half of their top placements. One thing leads to another, and the combination usually leads to a third: the exercise, plus the right diet, and—as the reward—peace of mind.

Start Daily Exercise!

Plenty of analysis points to how consistent exercise is beneficial for health of both body and soul. It:

- increases calorie burning which helps maintain body weight
- counteracts metabolic syndrome and diabetes
- increases HDL (high-density lipoprotein) good cholesterol
- counteracts bad fat (long-chain fatty acids)
- counteracts a long line of illnesses such as heart attacks, stroke, depression, some types of cancer, joint inflammation, and injuries caused by falls
- releases hormones and other substances that increase mental well-being
- increases enthusiasm and energy toward daily work tasks
- improves sleep

Just walking or riding the bicycle to work, instead of using the car, makes a big difference. Let your employer "offer exercise"—use the stairs instead of the elevator. It is also important to do your household chores yourself; cleaning windows and gardening offer plenty of exercise. Become a role model for your neighbors. Show them that you can do things yourself.

Brisk walking (speed walking) can be additional exercise; as can running, biking, dancing, badminton, tennis . . . it is difficult to point to one exercise as better than any other. It is important that you enjoy what you do. Taking pleasure in your activity ensures a good outcome.

TRAINING RESULTS CAN'T BE STORED

Your body can't store the results from training. The results are fleeting and need to be recaptured regularly each week.

To get the wished-for effect from exercise, you have to put in a substantial amount of effort. You need to become breathless and, preferably, start to perspire at least between the shoulder blades. A leisurely walk with the family dog doesn't really count here. Although it might benefit health, playing golf isn't likely to take enough exertion.

During the training, or at least part of it, the basic rule is to ensure that the pulse is properly elevated to at least 75 percent of maximum heart rate. It is extremely desirable to not only exercise the skeletal muscle, but also the most important muscle in the body—the heart—as well as our breathing apparatus, the lungs.

MAXIMUM HEART RATE IS NOT STATIC—IT CHANGES WITH NEEDS

A small child records a maximum heart rate of 225 heartbeats a minute. This will decrease by approximately 1 beat per year through their lifetime. This means that a seventy-five-year-old usually has a maximum heart rate of not much in excess of 150 heartbeats and needs to strive for a training pulse of approximately 120 heartbeats per minute. However, today there are many fit older persons who show higher maximum heart rate and therefore can train at a higher maximum rate. There are sophisticated measuring instruments you can attach to your chest to measure beats, and you can use telephone apps to register the beats and so on.

Here is a good basic rule for two people running or taking a *brisk* walk together: "You should barely be able to carry on a conversation with your training buddy, and if you can sing, your speed is too slow."

Don't forget that each age-group has its own needs.

CHILDREN UNDER 5 YEARS: It's sufficient for them to play, preferably outside, approximately three hours a day.

5 TO 18 YEARS: It is recommended that this group, where each individual child grows significantly during the period, gets at least one hour of intensive daily physical activity. This should be supplemented three times a week with specially organized activities like bicycling, soccer, or dance.

ADULTS (18 TO 64 YEARS): Recommended amount of exercise for this age-group is somewhat less than for adolescents. The training can be a bit less intensive, but still at least half an hour (½ hour) five days a week—this preferably includes interval training and/or speed changes.

OLDER (65 YEARS AND OLDER): The longer the elderly can continue middle-age-mode exercise the better. The more you exercise as you age, the more it contributes to counteracting disease and premature aging.

It is important that the daily exercise is done a few hours after a meal—preferably in the morning (after breakfast if you eat this). Studies have actually shown if someone has just eaten, and there are lots of antioxidants in the body, it can counteract health benefits from the exercise.

This kind of timing is not as important in competitions where long-term goals are not the main purpose. A copious amount of antioxidants might even be a great advantage. It is a well-known fact that endurance sports have certain short-term disadvantages. The competitor's immune system is depleted shortly after the effort, and the individual often catches cold.

DISADVANTAGE WITH OVERAMBITIOUS ATHLETICS

A word of warning here concerning children and young girls.

It is not unusual for 8- to 10-year-olds to train too hard. Training up to thirty hours per week might occur, but responsible physicians warn against this. It can cause serious consequences, both long and short term, for the health of children. It is noted that performance pressure in children's athletics today is increasing both from trainers and misguided overly ambitious parents who dream that their child will become the new Zlatan [Swedish soccer player] or Kalla [Swedish cross-country skier]. Marita Haringe, a specialist in gymnastic injuries at CIFA, the center for athletic injury research and education, is one of several who has commented on the unacceptably high level of injuries in certain sports.

The well-known physician to Olympic athlete Klas Österberg summed up the debate in one sentence: "Children should play, not train hard."

The disadvantages of overambitious athletics have been remarked upon in the medical literature, describing how a phenomenon called the female athlete triad syndrome is gaining traction among young gymnasts and dancers. This is a combination of disordered eating, amenorrhea and, despite training so hard, osteoporosis (loss of bone density, demineralization of the skeleton). Research shows that it might even be as many as five different negative manifestations—a pentad. Observations suggest that in this group type 2 diabetes can debut more often and earlier in life (early-onset diabetes), in addition to cardiovascular disease (early-onset coronary heart disease).

Unacceptably high incidents of stress fractures have been reported among, for instance, high school students in the United States who train too vigorously.

It has also been suggested that top athletes, who later in life retire from sports, have a higher frequency of illness when they age than athletes who train less hard. However, so far there has been little evidence to support this claim.

EXERCISE: RUN FROM ILLNESS

Well-adapted exercise shows unique properties that work as prevention for various serious illnesses. Here are a few examples:

Alzheimer's disease. Several publications indicate that a multitude of daily activities can strongly counteract the development of the illness. The described important goal is to fill the day with different social activities for the targeted group. At least six different studies have concentrated on the importance of exercise for Alzheimer's disease sufferers.

One reported effect is a delay in the illness' further development. Similar effects have been observed in other neurodegenerative diseases. Exercise is given extra importance for promoting calmer and better sleep for Alzheimer's disease and Parkinson's disease patients who often suffer from sleep disorders.

ADHD. A recently performed analysis of children who were "worn out" with sports (here it was table tennis) showed considerable improvements in many ways, for instance, better sleep and less "unruliness."

Diabetes. Elevated postprandial hyperglycemia is perhaps the most significant risk factor for increased illness and premature death in diabetes. Several studies have shown intensive exercise to be a powerful preventive measure here.

Breast cancer. Development of breast cancer, just as in Alzheimer's disease, is in part associated with bad dietary habits in childhood. The problems are directed to the consumption of dairy products as well as to obesity and a lack of exercise. It has been proven without a doubt today that regular exercise decreases the risk for certain cancers, and breast cancer is among them.

Treatment results in breast cancer patients have shown to improve when it is combined with regular exercise.

Prostate cancer. Studies show that using a diet dominated by raw and fresh foods can halt the progress of prostate cancer. This diet also managed to normalize the grading test of the cancer's progression.

The number of times an activity is performed and the level of exertion decide the achieved result. The very best result was reached when an activity was carried out more than three hours a week and at a speed of 3.11 mph (5 km per hour).

EXERCISE IS NOT ENOUGH TO FIGHT OBESITY

Before we start in on diet and weight in connection with exercise:

Remember that exercise on its own is never effective in the fight against obesity!

Two and one-quarter pounds (1 kg) body fat is about 9,000 calories. If you're overweight by 44 to 66 pounds (20–30 kg) the task of trying to "exercise fat away" becomes Herculean. A serious change in diet is necessary for success.

"Two and one-quarter pounds (1 kg) of body fat is about 9,000 calories."

The examples below show how many hours of normal daily activities are needed to burn 2¼ pounds (1 kg) of body fat.

Sleep—rest	(65 calories/hour)	134 hours
Watching television	(70 calories/hour)	128 hours
Office work	(85 calories/hour)	105 hours
Quick walk/brisk walking	(400 calories/hour)	23 hours
Cycling/spinning	(600 calories/hour)	15 hours
Running	(650 calories/hour)	14 hours
Swimming	(690 calories/hour)	13 hours
Hard manual labor	(700 calories/hour)	13 hours

The Highway to Fitness

We have already broached the subject of obesity and being overweight; not least how eating in the Western world has degenerated into a harmful fat and sugar intake compared to the Stone Age population's lean and green nourishment with a 80/10/10 diet makeup.

I don't enjoy sharing even more information about overweight and obesity, and it probably isn't encouraging for my readers either. But the starting position is dismal! What has happened and is happening with our dietary habits and our food industry is quite simply a very disturbing chapter. What is even worse is this: according to all prognosis it will only get worse as the rest of the world adjusts itself to our Western lifestyle—lots of stress, little exercise, and atrocious dietary habits. Don't shoot the messenger. I'm only telling it as it is.

"Obesity is caused by inflammation, and everything that causes inflammation effectively contributes to obesity."

Face the facts head-on when it comes to form and fitness: If you eat far too much fat and sugar, and also overeat, how will you manage to achieve good physical fitness?

However, we do have to point out that it isn't *only* too little exercise or too much food that makes you overweight. Far from it! Obesity is caused by inflammation, and everything that causes inflammation effectively contributes to obesity. A major problem is that obese individuals basically have a completely different microbiome marked by less of the good bacteria and much more of the illness-generating bacteria. These deliver more of the inflammation-provoking toxins like bacterial endotoxins to the body. The individuals also lack, as already mentioned, nearly all of many good bacteria.

The solution is to follow my twelve commandments with an additional "intestinal makeup" with efficient anti-inflammatory bacteria, like my research favorites *Lb plantarum* and *Lb paracasei*. These have shown themselves to be able to keep away antibiotic-resistant groups of bacteria.

Obesity will also be generated if you more or less completely "snuff out" the inflammation—something that is often seen in individuals who take strong anti-inflammatory drugs like cortisone, NSAIDs, and certain cytostatics.

CALORIE-DENSE FOOD IS THE MAIN REASON FOR OBESITY

In the chapter "Exchange the Farmer's Food for the Gardner's" beginning on page 108, you can read that it is mainly the food produced by agriculture—foods often refined and calories condensed through many industrial processes—that is the reason for our obesity and obesity-related illnesses.

The main culprits are sugar and sugar-like foods such as bread (even dark), pizza, warm root vegetables, pasta, and cooked refined white rice. Among the worst are the industrially baked gluten-free breads made from calorie- and starch-rich potato and corn starch flours that are nutritionally poor but cheap to use. Most of the vegetables we eat have been bred to give better harvests (more calories). Some are produced purely to up the profitability, through GMO (genetically modified organisms) which also contributes to making us both obese and ill.

It doesn't help to go vegetarian or vegan to counteract this. Cooking the sugar beet, sugarcane, or corn exactly like we prepare potatoes and other root vegetables in our own kitchens produces sugar. In reality, this actually adds nearly as much sugar, and sometimes even more, as store-bought items.

> "Limit or eliminate the consumption of long-chain fats: pork fat, beef fat (tallow) and oils such as olive oil, canola oil, and sunflower oil. Replace them with medium-chain fats like coconut oil and avocado oil."
>
> FROM MY TWELVE COMMANDMENTS FOR OPTIMAL HEALTH. P. 74

People also eat far too many long-chain fats, most of them coming from beef, pork, and dairy products. I have mentioned the bad qualities of these fatty acids in several instances, especially their inability to efficiently transform into energy. It is also through overconsumption of these fats that the earlier described postprandial inflammation enters the picture.

ADIPOSE TISSUE—THE BODY'S GARBAGE CAN

When the burden of chemicals, pharmaceuticals, hormones, microbes, bacterial toxins like endotoxins, uremic toxins, and a variety of toxic plastics becomes too heavy, the body struggles to get rid of it all. It then chooses to lock the toxins in the body's adipose tissue. A recently performed examination shows that obese individuals have two to three times the amount of chemical toxins stored in their adipose tissue compared to slim individuals.

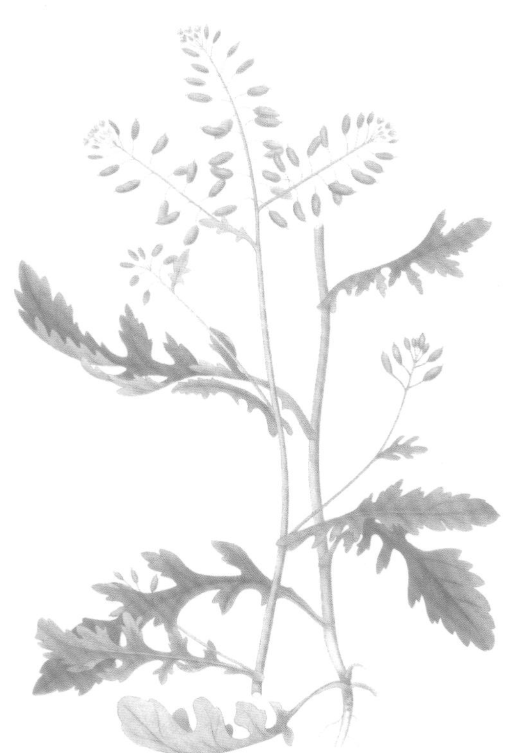

Environmental toxins arrive for instance with foods stored in plastic packaging. (Even food seemingly wrapped in paper has actually come into contact with plastic if the paper has a plastic lining.) We have long known that plastic migrates to other substances. It was observed about fifty years ago that plastic moved into plasma used for blood transfusions when the plasma was stored in plastic bags. I suspect this is the case today, too.

An unfortunate result of lots of "garbage" in the adipose tissue is the body reduces fat metabolism. This becomes slower and more ineffective when it is fully occupied with protecting the rest of the organs from toxins. As a consequence, weight loss becomes more difficult.

"THE DEADLY QUARTET"

Scientists in the United States, Canada, and Germany recently studied the mortality risk of various manifestations of disease. Instead of looking at different illnesses, they looked at mortality for different symptoms. As expected, smoking took first place; although with a slim margin as hypertension looked nearly as dangerous, followed by obesity. However, in 2017 obesity surpassed smoking as the leading cause of mortality.

Alcohol abuse arrives in tenth place, and the collective mortality risk of symptoms two to nine—all results of excessive consumption of the Western diet—is actually many times the total risk from smoking and alcohol.

Scientists today talk about the deadly quartet, that is, the four symptoms that collectively contribute to the highest risk for premature death: considerable obesity, hypertension, elevated blood glucose, and elevated blood lipids.

The Swedish researcher Eskil Kylin was the first (in 1923) to point out the risk from the symptoms of "dysfunction" in the body's metabolism: abdominal obesity, hypertension, abnormal blood lipids, lowered glucose tolerance, reduced HDL cholesterol, and an elevated level of uric acid in the blood. Today the combination is known as "metabolic syndrome."

Vitamin D deficiency also contributes to inflammation and obesity—even your mother's lifestyle, a subject discussed more in chapter 12.

Too much of pro-inflammatory proteins, both as supplements and/or as food ingredients (for example, gluten and casein) as well as pharmaceuticals, contribute also to increased inflammation. Poor circadian rhythm (poor sleep, day rhythm) with late nights and shift work or a detrimental lifestyle that might follow smoking cessation or too little attention to giving organs a rest. A typical example of the latter is snacking.

Reward Yourself with Stress Control

I personally felt an inner peace once I decided to choose health, both through diet and exercise.

"For whosoever hath, to him shall be given . . ." according to the Gospel of Matthew. A bit of both positive and negative truth there. If an inner peace can replace a markedly stressed frame of mind—both in brain and intestines—then there are plenty of health benefits to reap!

THE DIRECT CONNECTION BETWEEN BRAIN AND INTESTINES

It is well documented that our brain and immune system, whether we're healthy or sick, constantly exchange information to help us feel our best. The concept of the gut-brain axis, an entirely new field of knowledge, is built on how our brain seems to have a complete branch in our digestive system. This signaling system becomes incredibly important when we are subjected to stress. Chronic stress is probably the most dangerous of all known causes of illness, perhaps even worse than a bad diet.

Stress liberates a whole host of hormones, neuropeptides, and other neurochemical products that have devastating effects on the important functions of the immune system. Nearly all of our body cells are sensitive to these. Our immune system cells and gut microbiome are especially harmed by stress-related neuro-hormones like adrenaline and noradrenaline. All lymphatic organs—such as the bone marrow, thymus, spleen, and lymph nodes—are rich in nerve fibers that send messages from the brain. This applies not least to our gut.

The different body organs communicate in lots of ways, but the brain directs most. Apart from the brain and adrenal glands, the colon is a main player in stress. The colon is special, because it is often the "programmer" that directs the immune system while at the same time it's the home to around 2¼ pounds (1 kg) to 4½ pounds (2 kg) of gut bacteria. The two-way signaling between brain and gut increases dramatically in stress. Communication paths are many: fiber (nerve) connected conversation (synaptic signaling = when communication happens through synapses), wireless communication (endocrine signaling = when communication happens with other cells through the circulatory system), and nearby communication (paracrine signaling = when communication is between nearby cells) and autocrine signaling when the cell produces substances that affect its own functions. It's reported that our gut is provided with at least 500 million nerve fibers that connect it directly to the brain.

Our gut bacteria is "showered" by stress hormones such as adrenaline, noradrenaline, and dopamine during physical and mental stress. This radically changes the pattern of our gut bacteria, which manages to banish the good bacteria and let the harmful bacteria more or less take over. Medical literature reports that "stress hormones," such as naturally occurring adrenaline, noradrenaline, and dopamine, as well as synthetic pharmaceuticals such as dobutamine and isoprenaline (an asthma drug), increase the growth of harmful bacteria and their level of virulence, sometimes as much as 100,000 times.

COMMUNICATION AMONG DIGESTIVE ORGANS, GUT FLORA, AND THE BRAIN

Endocrine, paracrine, neurocrine, and inflammation-related communication > 500 million nerve fibers

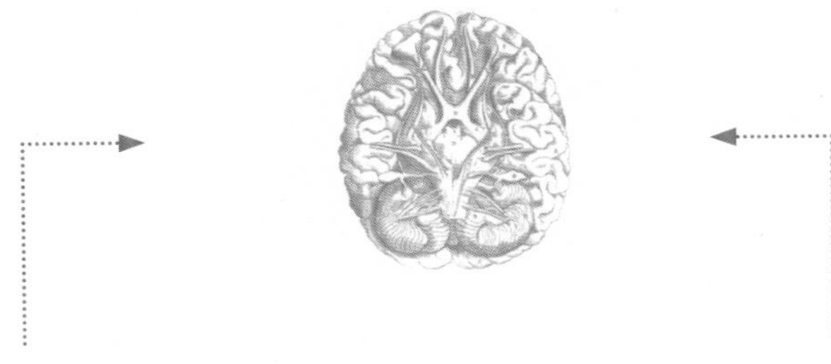

SYSTEMIC COMMUNICATION
HPA axis (hypothalamic-pituitary-adrenal—the "stress axis")
Neurotransmitters
Bacterial metabolites
Cytokines

COMMUNICATION
via NERVE FIBERS
Vagus nerve
Sympathetic nervous system

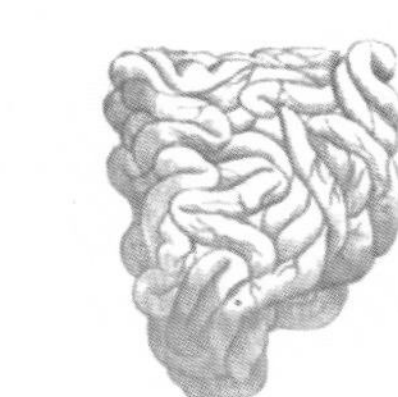

Source: Mayer, E. A.

Mental Stress Ruins the Digestion

It is well known that mental stress can lead to extensive problems and often to significant digestive and gut problems. For example, one of the most widespread diseases, IBS (irritable bowel syndrome) is strongly associated with psychological stress and bad gut flora.

Comprehensive studies done on astronauts, who are seen as living with more or less permanent stress, show an extensive and serious degradation of the gut flora and a strong reduction of bacteria (primarily lactobacillus and bifidobacteria) which might be in probiotics—and which is included in my latest synbiotics composition. A catastrophic increase of harmful bacteria was also noted in these groups.

Microbiome in university students were also studied during exam periods and in athletes who practice very strenuous sports. Many lose a large portion of their microbiome and immune system during especially stressful periods. They also frequently fall ill during these times, not uncommonly with serious infections.

It's my belief and hope that an intense reconditioning of the gut by synbiotics, that is, an addition of a combination of prebiotic fibers (food for the bacteria) and healthy bacteria, will minimize this risk.

THE DANGEROUS POTBELLY

Stress is extra dangerous if an individual is obese and especially if it's accompanied by a lot of abdominal fat (i.e., a "potbelly"). "potbelly". Stress brings multiple risks for acute cardiovascular disease, a cerebral hemorrhage for instance. Normally we should only have about 1 fl ounce (25 ml) fat on the intestines and the mesentery. That's what we believe our ancestors had. Modern studies have reported that some people showed an incredible 1½ gallon (6 liters) of fat in the abdomen.

Stress "ditches" large amounts of fat into the blood together with pro-inflammatory and pro-coagulant substances. In difficult cases, these can increase up to a thousandfold and will then accumulate an enormous fat collection in the liver, create insulin resistance, and induce a slew of diseases. You'll find a summary in the

METABOLIC SYNDROME IS THE GATEWAY TO OTHER CHRONIC DISEASES

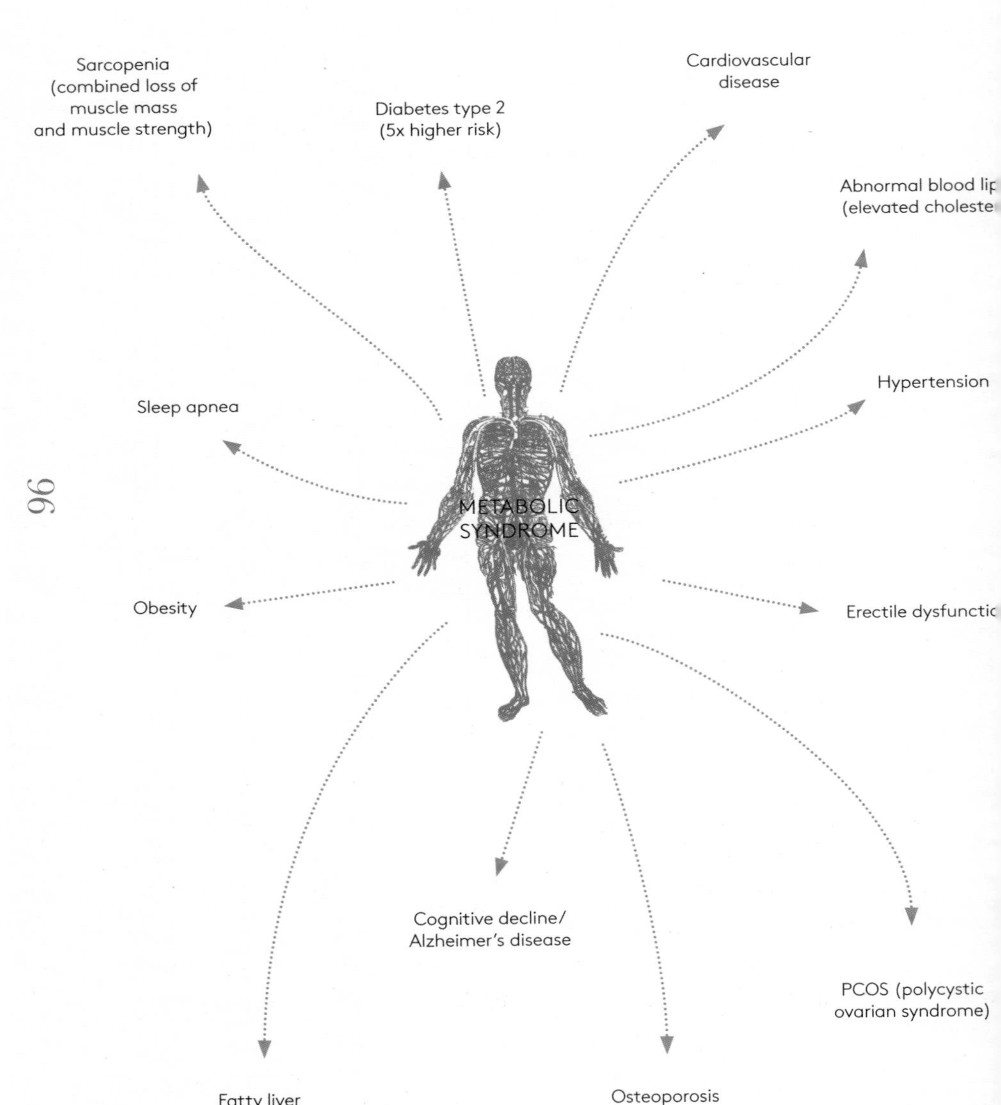

diagram to the left: cardiovascular disease, elevated cholesterol levels (dyslipidemia), hypertension, erectile dysfunction, PCOS, which means many ovarian cysts (polycystic ovarian syndrome), cognitive decline, osteoporosis, fatty liver, all-over obesity, sleep apnea, loss of muscle mass and strength (sarcopenia), and type 2 diabetes.

BETTER REWARD THAN CHIPS AND CANDY?

We have now touched on the three basic pillars of my method: The Anti-Inflammatory Diet Solution. Look at them as the three legs of a three-legged stool: it will topple over if you remove a leg. This applies not least to the leg I call stress control.

My belief is that the Western dietary garbage culture creates a free-floating anxiety in the individual. Apart from that, the food also creates a true physical stress in the body. It eases the acquired mental stress to have it out with your bad habits! I have seen many examples of this over the years.

It is high time that we stopped regarding excessively fatty and sweet foods, chips, and candy as rewards. Rewards? For whom? No, it is stress control that rather deserves the name!

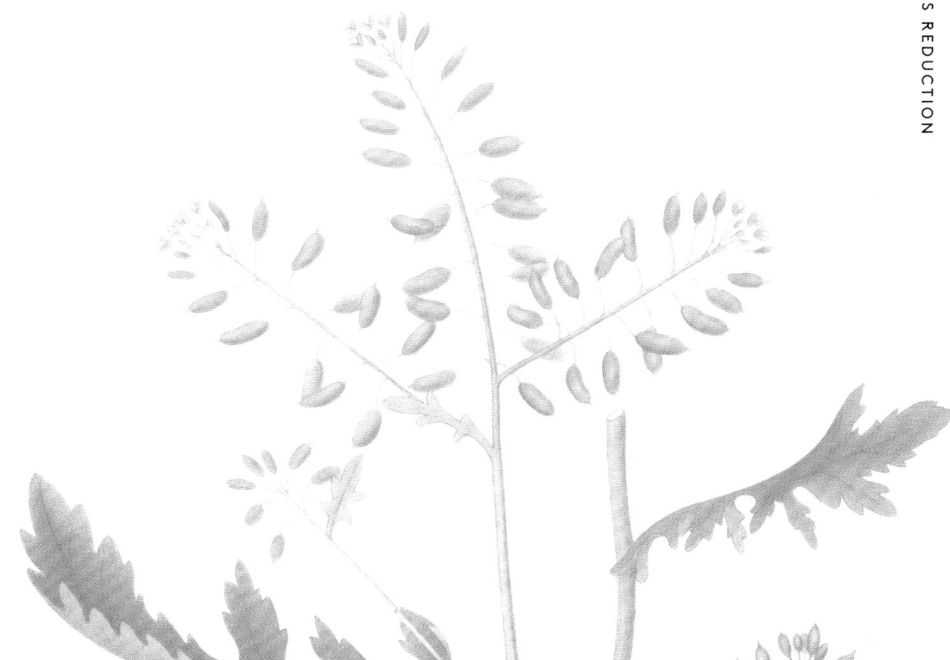

Carnivore, Vegetarian, or Vegan?

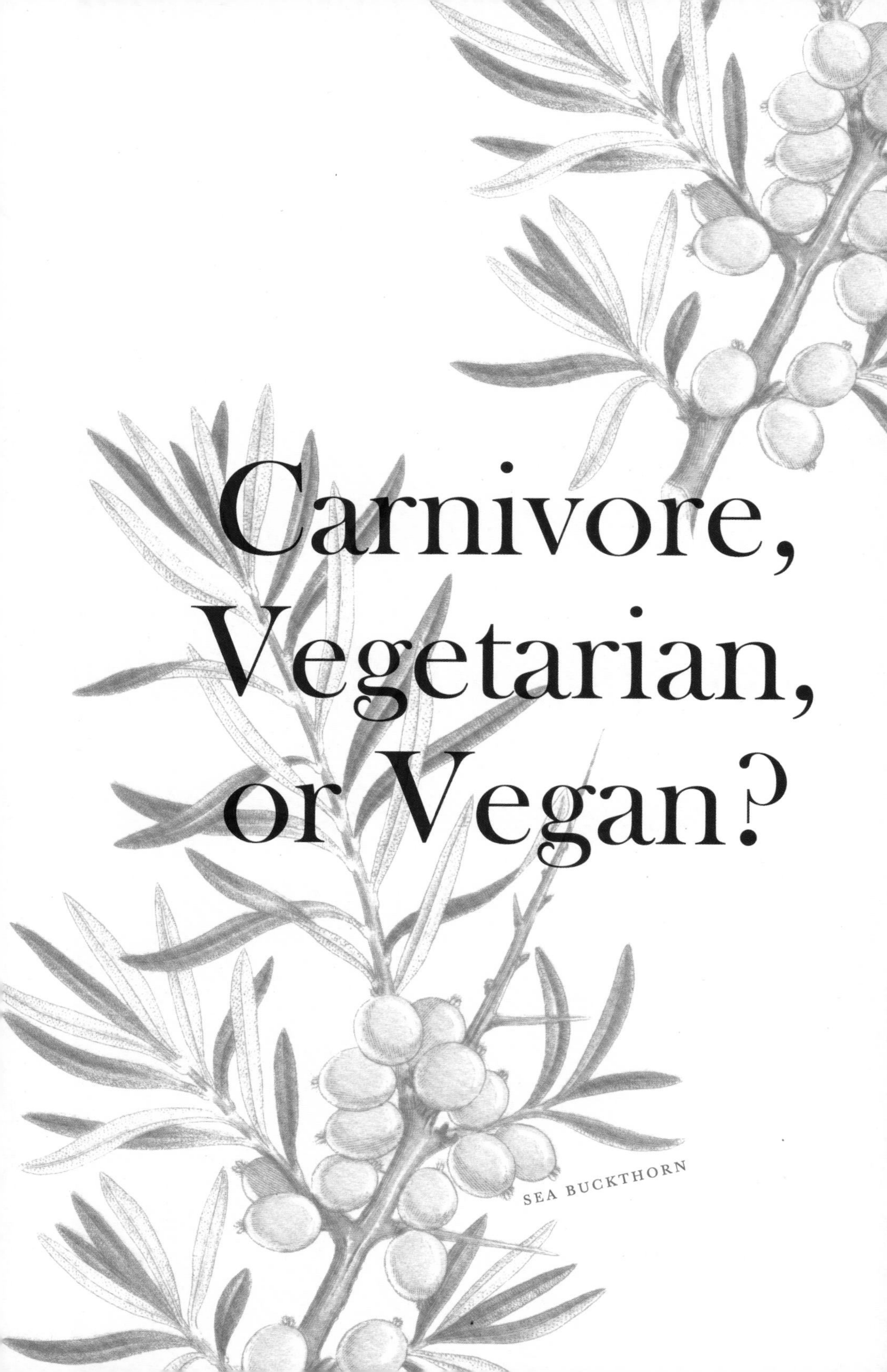

SEA BUCKTHORN

05

What suits your lifestyle best—being carnivore, vegetarian, or vegan? It is amazing to see how many who follow my work, especially among the younger generation, are profoundly engaged in this question. Many, but not all, avoid meat altogether.

I am glad to help you along if you're hesitant. If you've decided to eat meat, what drawbacks can you avoid if you choose and handle the meat correctly?

I will also explain a bit about what animal husbandry and meat production looks like from a global community perspective.

CONSUMPTION OF MEAT and processed meat products increased dramatically during the twentieth century. During the last fifteen years it has increased by more than 50 percent, although in Sweden it did decrease somewhat in 2017.

Large investigations show detrimental effects caused by high meat consumption.

Sweden's consumption of meat measures above the average EU (European Union) consumption, but there are countries with both higher and lower consumption than the Swedish.

Swedes consumed more than 33 pounds (15 kg) of meat above what the average EU citizen used in 2016. The biggest difference was seen in beef, where the Swedes ate more than 33 pounds (15 kg) more per person and per year. However, the average EU citizen consumed just as large amounts of pork as the average Swede.

The interest for a diet without elements of animals or animal products is actually increasing, which is encouraging. Comparison

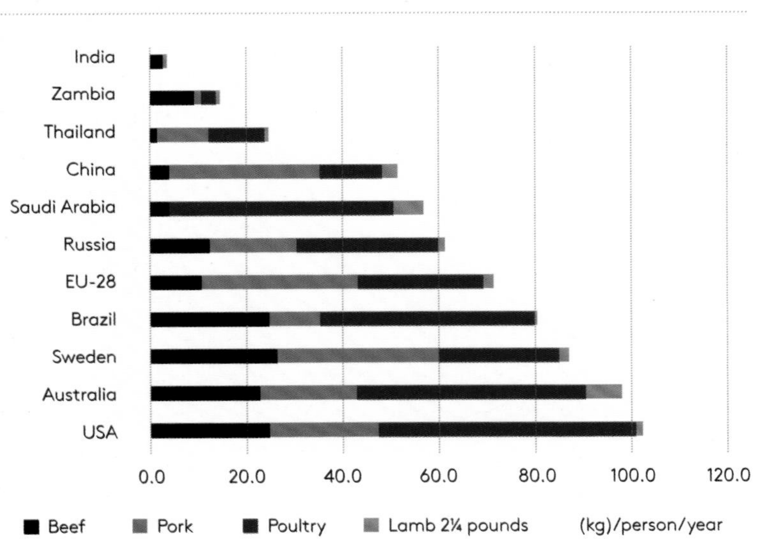

Source: The Swedish Board of Agriculture (2018)

between the average EU consumption and the average among the rest of the world's countries shows a big difference. For example, India's meat consumption is very low, while in the United States it is well above the average. The World Health Organization (WHO) recommends a meat consumption of not more than ¾ pound (350 g) a week. Several countries' food administrations have chosen to follow this guideline.

Vegetarians Who Disappeared . . .

There was a group of people who lived in Sweden in the middle of the 1900s calling themselves "raw fooders," or sometimes also "Waerlanders" after their leader Are Waerland.

This group has more or less disappeared by now. There are probably many reasons for this. They added a lot to their lifestyle, which was often not scientific; and it was sometimes even unhealthy. Eventually, it was evident that the Waerlanders' health or life span was in fact inferior to that of the average Swede. Perhaps the reason was the majority of the group replaced lean meat in their diet with large quantities of eggs and cheese?

Current studies show that vegans (they don't eat meat or dairy) are 20 percent healthier than meat eaters. Vegans also have a significantly lower accumulation of AGE and ALE than meat eaters.

Lacto-vegetarians (they add dairy) and ovo-lacto vegetarians (apart from dairy, they also add eggs), however, actually have an inferior health profile compared to meat eaters.

Several studies through the years have shown that vegetarianism is not a good middle-of-the-road solution. Vegetarianism was already questionable in the past, as the diet was often based on too much bread, cooked vegetables, root vegetables, and similar foods. Later studies have failed to show any special dramatic advantage from adapting to a vegetarian diet; in fact, quite the opposite. The eventual advantages that might have been observed were too small to warrant it to be "worth it" (i.e., go for a more radical change of lifestyle).

A lot points to the fact that it is more important to avoid or to greatly reduce the consumption of dairy products rather than meat. Even meat should be eaten with great moderation (we'll return to this later on).

. . . and Today's Winning Raw Fooders

At the same time, as many more people consistently left vegetarianism for raw food, lots of great benefits have become evident.

As a keen dairy-milk-refusing raw fooder, I happily note that you have to be a bit of a fundamentalist if you want to reach the desired results. As I also eagerly promote daily exercise, the result of this study is also gratifying:

A renowned American investigation compared twenty-one vegans (no meat, no dairy, no eggs) who lived for two years on raw food against twenty-one endurance runners (marathon, triathlon, and such trials) who on average ran forty-eight miles (77 km) a week for at least five years, as well as twenty-one sedentary subjects (the ones who couldn't care less, eat Western junk diet, and don't exercise).

Those who exercised were healthier than those who didn't, but the vegans showed the absolute best values for, for instance, blood pressure, blood glucose, insulin resistance, and circulating harmful fats.

Most startling, to my mind, is that in the raw food group you could see that the width of the artery to the head, the carotid artery, was half the width of that observed in those we call "couch potatoes"—the group practicing a Western lifestyle. The difference in BMI (body mass index) between the groups was very evidently to the raw fooders' advantage, and to the couch potatoes' disadvantage.

It is interesting to note that the vegans actually consumed a lot less energy—on average less than 2,000 calories/24 hours while the endurance athletes consumed an average of 2,300 calories, and the "couch potatoes" more than 2,600 calories. The intake of carbohydrates was quite similar between the groups. The big difference lay in that the vegans' carbohydrates were never heated, always left raw. Another big difference was the vegans ate twice as much fiber,

50 percent more fat (overwhelmingly good fats), as well as significantly more "wholesome" salt (potassium), and less than half as much protein and "harmful" salt (sodium). In addition, the vegans consumed hardly any trans fats. The intake was only a fraction of what the other groups consumed—0.014 ounce/day (0.4 g/day) compared with ⅕ ounce/day (5.3 g) and ¼ ounce/day (5.9 g).

Unhealthy Feed, Sick Animals

Let's return to the question of meat eating to look at the problems today's animal production brings.

Our most common farm animals, the ruminants—cows, sheep, and goats—are made to feed on grass and bushes, just like pigs were meant to live off roots. Today's farming practices have changed to become more efficient. This is especially relevant for cows and pigs, which are now eating concentrated feed and grains, having incalculable negative effects for both the environment and our health.

In the past, the ruminants had an important part to play in people's households. They could transform non-edibles for humans (grass and bushes) into edible foods. Today the ruminants instead compete in a major way with us for the same food that we ourselves eat. This can be seen as a serious threat, especially as a cow eats just about the same amount as ten humans. There are about half as many ruminants as humans on earth today. What about in thirty years, when it's estimated that we will be equal in number. How will the world's diet look then?

We know that it takes about 5,283 gallons (20,000 liters) to produce 2¼ pounds (1 kg) of beef. For vegetables, it's less than a twentieth of this for each 2¼ pounds (1 kg). Much points to water shortages causing tomorrow's headache. Today's farming, with its high proportion of ruminant-based food production, doesn't look promising for the long term seen from that perspective. The reorganization of animal husbandry has been very economically successful, but it has had immense effects on both environment and health.

In 1850, a cow gave on average about 1½ quarts (1½ l) of milk a day. Today it gives more than twenty times as much. A pig needs two years to reach 220 pounds (100 kg) if it eats a species-appropriate diet. Today's factory farm achieves the same result in less than a quarter (¼) of that time. The cow, just like the pig, develops during this intensive force feeding in principle the same diseases as humans. The illnesses seldom have time to develop fully as both cows and pigs have been removed from the production line before this.

Research shows that calves that are brought up mainly on their mother's milk have, within a few months, developed precursors (glucose intolerance and insulin resistance) to diabetes.

It is also well known that our pigs suffer from constant loose stools, have a great tendency to develop gastric ulcers, abdominal adhesions, ileus, and infections. Factory-farmed cows and pigs suffer from lifelong chronically elevated inflammation. Transmission to the individual that eats the meat and drinks the milk, unfortunately to date, has not been fully investigated.

RAIN FOREST DEFORESTATION, GREENHOUSE EFFECT

Each day tens of thousands of acres of rain forest are being devastated under the pretext the land is needed to produce food for humans. However, the real truth is, in the last fifty years all newly cleared acreage is wholly allocated to production of fuel and animal feed. This goes primarily to farm animals but also to pets.

Farming with its animal husbandry causes overall 50 percent more greenhouse gases than the collective traffic on all roads, rail, in the air, and on the sea. The cows on the earth produce 50 percent more negative greenhouse gases than road traffic. What is even worse is you cannot regulate a cow's burps and farts like you can the discharge from a car's motor exhaust.

Even the pet population's effect is substantial. Compare a cow, which gives approximately eight gallons (30 liters) of milk daily while using up resources equivalent to that of twenty "average" human beings, with a dog that uses up the equivalent amount of four "average" humans. The earth's population of 500 million dogs eat as much meat as two billion humans. It has been calculated that a large dog uses as much of the earth's resources as a big-city jeep that is driven 1,000 miles a year.

I personally eat nowhere near ¾ pound (350 g) of meat a week. The reason is to look after the environment. It is extremely inefficient and uneconomical having the field's harvest first go through an animal stomach before it is consumed. If this didn't happen, nearly three times as many people could be fed.

"So—thank you, all vegans, for your contribution to the environment!"

Merely a few percent of the energy produced from the fields is left after a meat animal has used up 85 percent (chicken) to 98 percent (beef) of the nutrition—to warm itself, among other things. This inefficiency is especially remarkable if you consider each year fifty-six billion animals are slaughtered purely to satisfy humanity's desire for meat. This number is estimated to double in the years up to 2050.

So—thank you, all vegans, for your contribution to the environment! In my opinion, there are enough reasons overall to warrant moderation in meat eating—and to instead choose fish.

PROCESSED MEAT IS THE VILLAIN

We are, without a doubt, eating far too much meat. It is imperative that consumption is dramatically reduced. The results from two important and very extensive studies show this.

In one study performed in North America, 37,698 men and 83,644 women were followed over a period of more than twenty-eight years. Among the meat eaters the number of "premature deaths" increased 13 percent, mainly for cancer and cardiovascular disease. If they consumed a lot of processed meat—bacon, sausage, meatballs, paté, etc.—the premature death frequency increased to

20 percent—in fact, more than one in five.

In the second study, completed in several European countries, 448,568 subjects were followed for thirteen years. Daily meat consumption resulted in an increase in mortality during the thirteen years the study went on. If the meat consumed was industrially processed (i.e., fried, grilled, smoked, or made into sausage or meatballs) even here "premature" death was prevalent. Even this study showed one in five subjects (20%). Additionally, risk for death due to cardiovascular disease was increased by 72 percent, death due to cancer by 11 percent.

Many point to the industrialized treatment as the biggest villain here, and that careful handling can reduce the health risks significantly when eating meat. However, remember that less harmful methods are not enough. Most important is that we dramatically reduce the amount of meat we eat.

Personal Answer about Meat Consumption

Do we eat meat or not, is one of the most frequent questions I receive personally.

The question is not that easy to answer. We are not total vegans in our family, mostly because the scientific proof is not in yet. As mentioned before, we eat very little meat. If you want to do like us, eat some meat from warm-blooded animals. It is perhaps a good idea to first choose among poultry and game, meat from grass-fed animals and grass- and bush-eating animals. When it concerns pork, choose pasture-raised, foraging root-eating animals. Plenty depends on what the animals are fed, how the meat is handled, and how much we consume. For us, this is what counts:

- The meat will come from animals fed the same food the species have lived on millions of years—a feed without addition of flour and sugar (concentrates)—which means that we prefer wild game. Unfortunately even game is given extra feed nowadays. It is often not grass and root vegetables, but grains (which is often cheaper).

- The meat can't be hung as long as is practiced today because even dead bacteria possess strong inflammation-provoking effects.
- It's also important for us that the meat, like other food, is not prepared over high heat (never seared, fried or grilled), just lightly cooked or even better, prepared in a low-temperature oven. This means at the most 158°F to 176°F (70°C to 80°C) for several hours (according to the "frozen lump" method).
- The meat counters teem with "bad" and cheap meat, but it is increasingly common in restaurants in the United States and in certain areas in Europe to talk about "only grass-fed meats" and "meat prepared in a slow oven." If this is difficult to find, we have to hope that meat from grazing areas, like South America's enormous pampas, comes from animals raised that way.

Limit the consumption of meat to at most 3/4 pound (300 g) a week. Avoid processed meat: smoked, fried, grilled, sausage, meatballs, hamburgers, and similar items. Also avoid meat from animals reared on concentrates. Look for grass-fed meat. Avoid farmed fish and look for wild-caught fish.

FROM MY TWELVE COMMANDMENTS FOR OPTIMAL HEALTH. P. 74

Exchange the Farmer's Products for the Gardener's

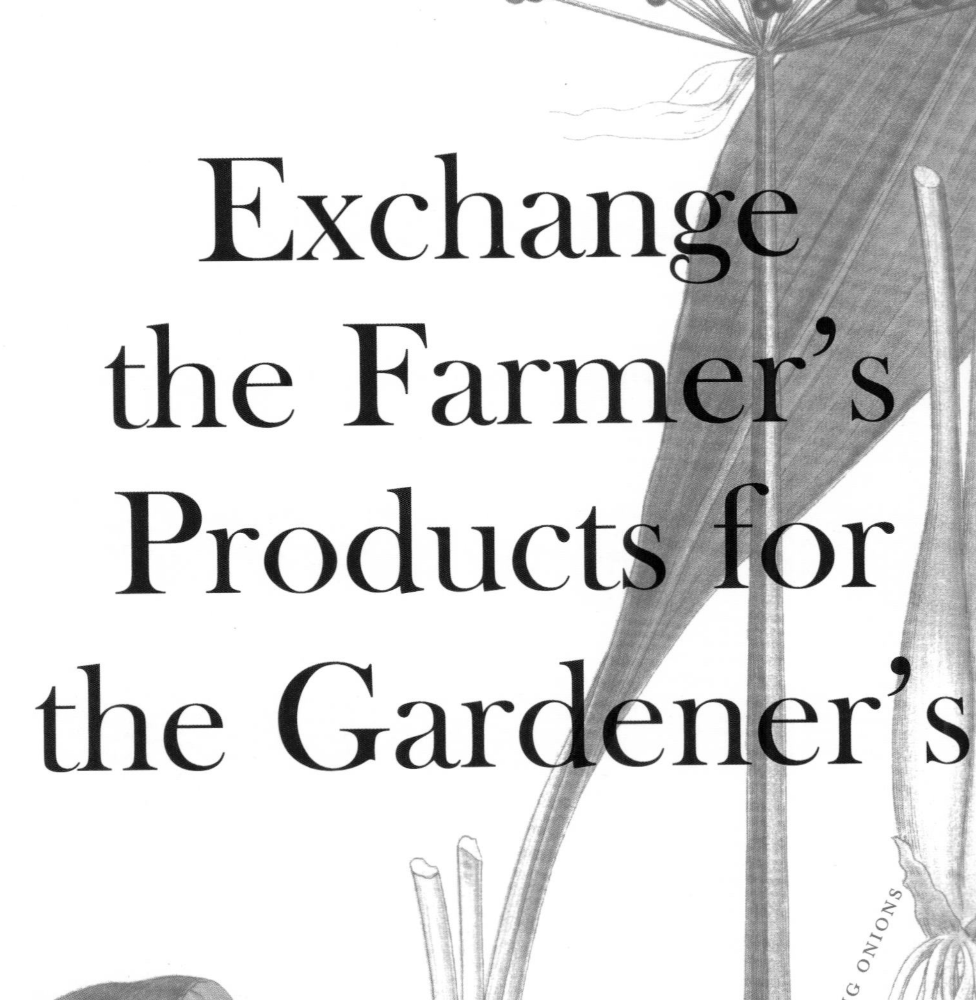
SPRING ONIONS

06

When I was a child everybody thought that there was nothing better than a glass of milk and a sandwich. The same pattern stands firm today even if it has been toned down somewhat. A popular café item today is a huge milk-dominated latte, together with a baguette or some other kind of large piece of—often white—bread. Cold cuts decorating it might be "cured" meats like salami or a dairy product like Brie cheese.

It is important to change ideas here, not only about the milk but also about meat products and the bread! It isn't just for us, the consumers, that a new way of thinking is important. It is equally important for people who raise the dairy animals and the farmer, who grows, produces, sells, and serves farm produce. Not least is this important for the ones deciding agricultural policies.

I HAVE NOW arrived at a purposely drastic conclusion that you might already have suspected:

Exchange the farmer's products for the gardener's!

I really don't want to harm the farmer. However, I am convinced that current animal husbandry and production of animal products, just like much of our current crops, need to be thoroughly evaluated and in many instances replaced.

We've already talked about *meat*. Let's continue by looking at the still-significant consumption of milk and dairy products in our part of the world.

Milk Does Not Make Bones Grow Stronger!

The consumption of dairy products per person per year in Europe increased steadily during more than a hundred years. However, during the last twenty years (imagine that!) consumption of milk and butter has had a dramatic downturn. For example, the consumption of butter has decreased nearly 50 percent. This has been observed in all of Europe and most notably in Sweden.

Research performed by Swedish scientists in six countries showed that the frequency of cardiovascular disease had decreased in five of these countries in parallel with the reduced consumption of dairy products.

Portugal, however, one of the countries that increased consumption of dairy products during this period, also showed a corresponding uptick in cardiovascular disease.

The findings speak loud and clear. It is better for heart and arteries to reduce the consumption of dairy products.

We know that the average consumption of cheese in Western Europe has increased worryingly during the last thirty years, from around 11 pounds (5 kg) to 44 pounds (20 kg) per individual and year.

Hormones, which we will return to shortly, follow the fat in the milk and are therefore found in abundance in butter and cheese. For instance, full-fat milk contains twice the amount of hormones as skim milk.

What is it that makes dairy products problematic—especially when eaten in excess?

IN THE MILK: SUGAR, CASEIN, BAD FATS . . .

What is common for dairy products is the large quantities of the sugars lactose and D-galactose.

Both lactose and D-galactose contribute strongly to increased inflammation in the body. In animal tests D-galactose has also been shown to cause, even in very low doses, tissue breakdown (especially in the nervous system), memory loss, premature aging, and shortened life span.

Dairy products also contain, apart from plenty of sugar, a large amount of the protein casein. Casein possesses strong inflammation-provoking properties that counteract growth/regeneration of good colon bacteria.

There are also plenty of saturated long-chain fatty acids in dairy products. These generate elevated blood cholesterol and risk factors for atherosclerosis later in life.

Only fats with less than twelve carbon atoms can go straight to the liver through the portal artery. Long-chain fatty acids, like "beef fats" and common cooking oils, are forced to take the long way to the liver via the lymphatic system and the general blood circulation. The disadvantage with this is the fats stay far too long in the circulation, often several hours, which makes the blood more viscous. These fats also slowly settle in the arterial walls. If any narrow passages exist, for example, in the heart or the brain's blood vessels, all this can cause an infarct, or brain hemorrhage. Also, one of the most important parts of the body's immune system, the luminal surface lining (the endothelium) of the vascular system becomes extremely strained. The immune cell macrophages become exceedingly vulnerable when they work hard to remove the fat from the blood.

There are also large amounts of heat-generated toxins that are especially present in dried milk. I have already mentioned Louis Camille Maillard, the Frenchman who discovered this in heated foods, and about the substances AGE and ALE that are so reminiscent of soot.

Pasteurizing (heating) of milk creates upward of a hundred of these toxic inflammation- and illness-generating substances.

HORMONAL CONFUSION

A balanced hormonal system is vital for our health and well-being.

Because of this, it is very worrying that today's dairy products contain such a large amount of hormones. Especially high elevated levels of the female sex hormone estrogen are found.

> "It's estimated that upward of 80 percent of the steroids humans ingest come from dairy products."

The insemination technique has resulted in that nearly all milk-producing cows are calving. This means that approximately 80 percent of all dairy products come from pregnant cows.

The result is, dairy products contain far too large amounts of hormones and growth factors that are really meant to get the calf to adult size and sexually mature within a year. However, they make the products highly problematic for human consumption.

The milk is thus riddled with hormones, everything from brain and pituitary gland hormones to hormones from the thyroid gland and gastrointestinal peptides. Above all, steroids like estrogen and progesterone, and even testosterone, are present. It's estimated that upward of 80 percent of the steroids humans ingest they get from dairy products.

In girls, this contributes to early breast development and ever earlier menstrual start and sexual maturity. The large amount of added hormones also affects expectant mothers' and boys' development negatively as they can contribute to, among other things, obesity and higher birth weights.

HIGH ESTROGEN LEVELS

Estrogen and growth factor content in milk appear to have increased in step with rationalization of milk production.

Researchers at the Institute for Risk Assessment Sciences (IRAS) at Utrecht University reported in 2007 very high doses of total estrogen in milk. There were considerably higher levels than we knew to date; and according to the authors, "dramatically more than observed earlier." A few months later, in a follow-up telephone call to the head of the institute, it appeared that the industry had reacted with total silence to hush up the result of the study.

The knowledge has, despite the silent treatment, contributed to a so-called hormone-free milk now being available in certain countries. They are also trying to reduce milk's pro-inflammatory properties by adding different substances.

To date, scientists have blamed the fat in dairy for the increased frequency of illness at higher consumption. The reason is probably just as much the hormones—and possibly a combination of the two.

DAIRY PRODUCTS AND CANCER

Forty years ago, Canadian researchers pointed out a clear connection between consumption of dairy products and the occurrence of breast cancer.

The connection showed breast cancer was highly concentrated in countries with elevated consumption of dairy products, and nearly wholly absent in countries with low consumption. The time wasn't right. Nobody took this observation seriously, and the industry did everything to keep milk's reputation wholesome. Several more decades had to pass, and hundreds of thousands more people had to die from breast cancer, before the world was ready to admit that there was a problem with dairy.

In Japan, prostate cancer frequency increased twenty-five-fold between 1948 and 1998; at the same time consumption of dairy products in the country increased 2,000 percent (still far lower than Sweden's consumption). Now the Chinese arrive in the picture. They lived for thousands of years with little or no consumption of dairy products, but are now striving to fully adopt the Western

BREAST CANCER MORTALITY IN A COUNTRY IN RELATION TO AVERAGE FAT CONSUMPTION IN THE SAME COUNTRY

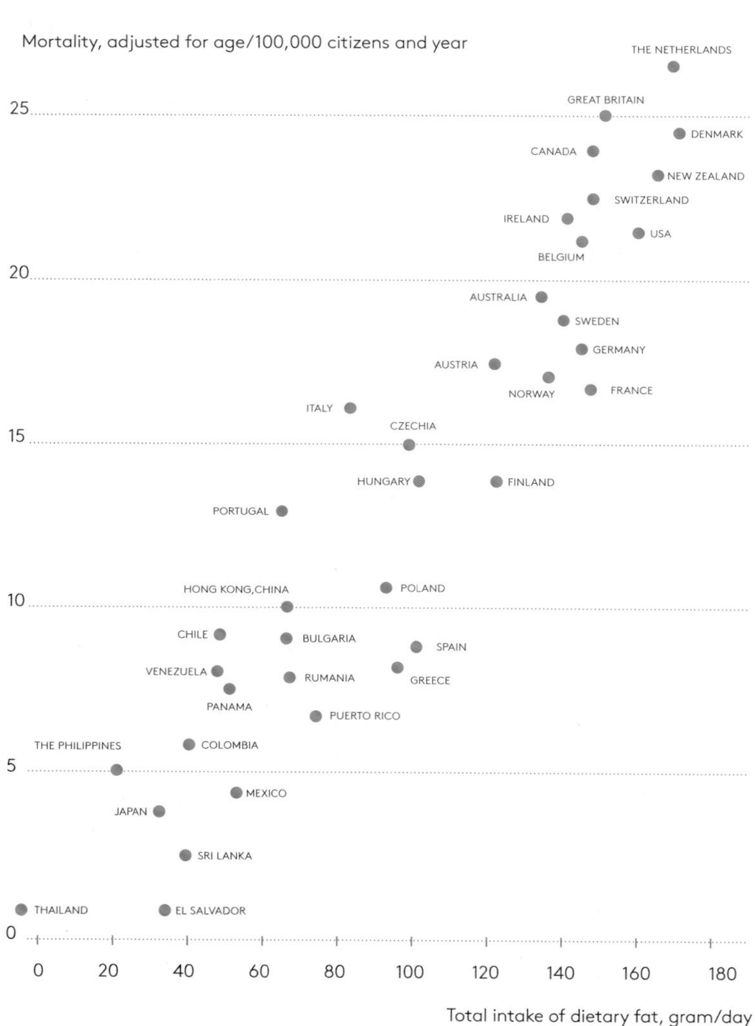

Source: Caroll, K. K., and Myles, I. A.

lifestyle. Their milk consumption is rising steeply, especially in the larger cities. This worries my Chinese colleagues who now see the incidence of breast and prostate cancer doubling every ten years.

A twenty-five-year Icelandic study of just over nine thousand men, of whom two thousand were afflicted with prostate cancer, showed those who consumed large quantities of milk in adolescence had approximately a 320 percent greater risk for developing prostate cancer than those who had consumed just a small amount.

Several cancers depend strongly on hormones for their emergence and growth—especially in the testicles, breast, prostate, ovaries, uterus, and colon. In higher doses, the above-named hormones are already known to promote inflammation in the body and diseases like cancer. Even illnesses other than cancer, everything from various autoimmune disorders to Parkinson's disease, show similar connections.

STOP PUTTING MILK ON A PEDESTAL!

Having studied the subject in depth, it's a mystery to me why cow's milk has achieved this exalted status. Perhaps we are confusing mothers milk's wholesomeness with the animal milk's unwholesomeness for humans? That's a major mistake if that is the case.

Many of us older folks remember the full-page advertisements featuring celebrities jumping for joy. The slogan was the same for all: "Milk builds strong bones!"

A robust Swedish investigation was published several years ago. For just over twenty years, it followed about 61,000 women and 45,000 men from Uppsala [a town in Sweden], Västmanland [a region in Sweden], and Örebro [a town in Sweden]. The individuals who consumed plenty of dairy products (milk, cheese, butter, and yogurt) showed a statistically important higher share of premature mortality. Not surprisingly, they also showed a higher incidence of fractures (i.e., signs of osteoporosis).

After approximately twenty years, 15,000 women were actually deceased and just over 17,000 had suffered some kind of bone fracture. Of the men who were followed, after eleven years about 10,000 out of the 45,000 were deceased and 5,000 had suffered a fracture.

We can toy with the idea that the Swedish farmers' output had been just as strictly supervised as the tobacco industry in the United States. There, the tobacco companies have regularly faced million-dollar fines for "deceptive marketing." The American government staked billions of dollars on alternative crops once it was obvious tobacco farming was in sharp decline. They assisted former tobacco farmers in cultivation of peanuts, peas, beans, etc.

But not in Sweden. The protective hand stays over the milk producers. Even though the figures are alarming, the dairy industry can feel secure; its products have had a firm place on a pedestal for hundreds of years that cannot be questioned.

> Reduce or eliminate all dairy products—especially butter, cheese and powdered milk.
>
> FROM MY TWELVE COMMANDMENTS FOR OPTIMAL HEALTH, P. 74

What Harm Has Bread Ever Done?

My essential view of most of the bread that we eat is that it is too calorific and its glycemic index is far too high. All too often I've felt compelled to inform happy sandwich-munchers that bread really is both too sweet and too poor nutritionally. It's often just empty calories.

Some bread has an even higher glycemic index than pure sugar. This applies also to gluten-free breads that are, in most cases, just pure garbage made from potato and corn flour.

On average, bread is also far too lacking in plant fiber. That's the reason why many become obese after having eaten too much bread over a prolonged period. Bread also contains gluten, which causes a problem for many more individuals than just gluten allergy sufferers.

To make matters worse, bread is heated to far too high temperatures, which leads to the formation of heat-created toxins. Sugar "marries" protein at as low a temperature as 176°F (80°C). Around a hundred heat-generated toxins have been identified in the last ten to fifteen years. We have already mentioned acrylamide as one of them. This is the toxin that halted the construction of the Halland (Swedish province) Tunnel for several years. The problem is that the acrylamide formation increased steeply after 275°F (135°C). Compare this to store-bought bread which is often baked at a temperature of up to 572°F (300°C) or more.

You'll find these toxins in especially large amounts in different kinds of chips, as well as in whey cheese and whey butter. Crispbreads and toast also contain large amounts; the heating and toasting multiply the acrylamide content at least tenfold.

GLUTEN—FORMERLY WALLPAPER GLUE

I sigh deeply sometimes when I reflect on how warped the Western dietary habits have become. A daily protein amount is around 1½ ounces to 2½ oz (40–70 g), but most Swedes eat four to five times that. Proteins are not something to be trifled with. Too large an intake of the wrong kinds of proteins can play havoc with our health. The already-named casein, the dominant protein in milk, is one; and gluten, which is found in grains like rye, barley and wheat, is another.

Everyday bread is gluten rich. The amount of gluten in bread has nearly multiplied twenty times since the use of our original grains. The reason is to get fast-rising bread. However, this is of no small importance! Bread is highly inflammation provoking and extremely harmful for our health—not just for the gluten-intolerant but also for all of us. The endemic disease IBS (irritable bowel syndrome) is strongly associated with gluten content in food.

Gluten doesn't just increase inflammation in the body—it also counteracts the regeneration of a healthy gut microbiome. Gluten has the same effect in the body as the potent bacterial endotoxin. 100 µg/ml gluten exerts the same inflammation producing effect as 10ηg/ml endotoxin (LPS—lipopolysaccharide). Classical experiments from seventy years ago showed that good gut bacteria didn't want to grow when they were exposed to gluten and casein.

"Gluten is worthless from a nutritional point of view."

Humans lived a gluten-free existence for the first 99.9 percent of their time on earth. It's suggested that once gluten was introduced into the daily diet a number of diseases made their debut, and the most gluten-sensitive population died off. Today's bread contains many times the amount of gluten compared to bread that was made with ancient grains.

Gluten is worthless from a nutritional point of view. The body can't break it down and cannot benefit from it as energy at all. The only value is in its capacity to make a dough rise quickly. Gluten is a glue, and its function is to seal the air bubbles inside the dough. Gluten was used for wallpapering in the past.

Scientific studies report in increasing numbers the connection between consumption of gluten and diseases like ADHD, arthritis, allergy, autoimmune disease, rheumatic illness, dementia, depression, diabetes, obesity, Grave's disease, IBS, IBD (inflammatory bowel disease, ulcerous colitis, and Crohn's disease), psoriasis, osteoporosis, schizophrenia, and different skin conditions, such as vitiligo (patches with loss of skin pigmentation).

Gluten consumption is associated in these studies with lethargy, fatigue, and low energy levels, while a gluten-free existence is associated with increasing energy and heightened enthusiasm.

ATHLETES CUT OUT GLUTEN

Top athletes already understand the benefit of cutting out gluten, and show noticeable difference in performances. It was reported that the majority of athletes followed gluten-free diets at the 2012 Olympic Games in London.

The top-seeded tennis players, Novak Djokovic and Andy Murray, both belong to the gluten-free top athletes. They blacklist many unhealthy foods including processed carbohydrates, lactose, and gluten, and report great positive effects from doing this.

In her forties and still among the world's elite marathon runners, Paula Radcliffe was asked what her secret is. She answered:

"I don't eat any dairy products or wheat and I don't use any anti-inflammatory pharmaceuticals."

More and more people join the circle of gluten-free athletes, and you'll find them in all sports today. There are many advantages in going gluten-free according to the elite athletes:

- blood glucose stays more level
- less inflammation in the body
- decreased joint and muscle pain
- increased energy and stamina
- improved digestion and improved energy uptake from the food
- decreased "rumbles and upsets in stomach" and bloating
- strengthened immune system
- decreased amount of infections, especially colds, the days after a competition
- lessens delayed muscle soreness and hastens the body's recuperation, especially in the muscles

As the athletes turn away from gluten, they abandon the old practice of carbohydrate loading based on consuming large quantities of processed carbohydrates. Fresh fruit and vegetables are increasingly replacing them.

If gluten fatigues, while gluten-free enhances energy and is good for athletes, then it ought to be good for schoolchildren as well.

Many Swedish children's diets consist of gluten, sugar, and dairy products. This actually contributes to tired children, creating a bad learning environment.

WILL "CORN-FREE" FOLLOW GLUTEN-FREE?

Gluten-free is often used in medicine, often as a "last resort." There are reports of epileptic adolescents who did not benefit from drug treatments, but when they went gluten-free the symptoms went away. Other reports exist about older individuals with forms of dementia other than Alzheimer's, who suddenly "cleared" mentally after gluten was removed from their diet.

I was especially impressed by a study done in 2003. Twelve out of fourteen patients with type 1 diabetes showed significantly improved insulin sensitivity after going gluten-free. These improvements disappeared completely, however, when they returned to their former eating habits after six months.

Similar experiences were reported after extensive studies of IBS and ADHD.

Recent animal tests show that mothers that have lived gluten-free during the pregnancy don't give birth to offspring with type 1 diabetes, and probably not other diseases within that family, like, for example, celiac disease.

Much suggests that we might arrive even further along in our quest for better health if we abstain from corn, which isn't only extremely calorific and obesity-promoting (one movie bag of popcorn contains, according to a recent British study, more than 1,000 calories). Corn also contains zein, a gluten-like substance that didn't receive much attention earlier. In animal studies, zein was shown to have more negative effects than both casein and gluten.

"Much suggests that we might arrive even further along in our quest for better health if we abstain from corn."

Divest Ourselves of Traditional Farming

I often feel embarrassed in international situations knowing our Swedish food culture remains as dietarily ignorant as it is currently.

Sometimes I've been forced to admit that two of the most renowned Swedish contributions to the international culinary scene are a sandwich and a glass of milk, and meatballs and mashed potatoes (often from desiccated and reconstituted potatoes). With our world-class chefs who often win international culinary competitions, surely we deserve to be known for something better?

I sometimes show a picture of a loaf of white bread, a banana, a bag of sugar, and a Snickers bar during a lecture. I then ask the audience which one they think contains the "most sugar," that is, has the highest glycemic index (GI). Just about everybody will point to the refined, white sugar. But no, that is not correct. It is actually the loaf of white bread that is highest on the GI index.

When asked to summarize my health advice in one sentence, my answer is usually the title of this chapter: Exchange the farmer's products for the gardener's.

As I've already mentioned, I wish the farmer well, at the same time that I wish he would retrain to become a market gardener! More than 90 percent of obesity is the result of traditional highly processed farm products, from grains to dairy products.

We can't blame the farmer because people routinely heat root vegetables. Nevertheless, it is a fact that the seven most serious warning signs of ill health are the result of eating too much of just the farmer's products:

- abdominal obesity/potbelly
- hypertension
- elevated blood fats (fats consisting of more than 12 carbon atoms)
- elevated blood glucose
- low good cholesterol
- elevated uric acid in the blood
- elevated inflammation—elevated C-reactive protein (CRP) in the blood

It's obvious that we need more healthy grains and daily beverages other than cow's milk. I want the farmers to join me in this endeavor.

Many interesting products are already under development for both farm and food markets.

The Body's Heart-Healthy Friends

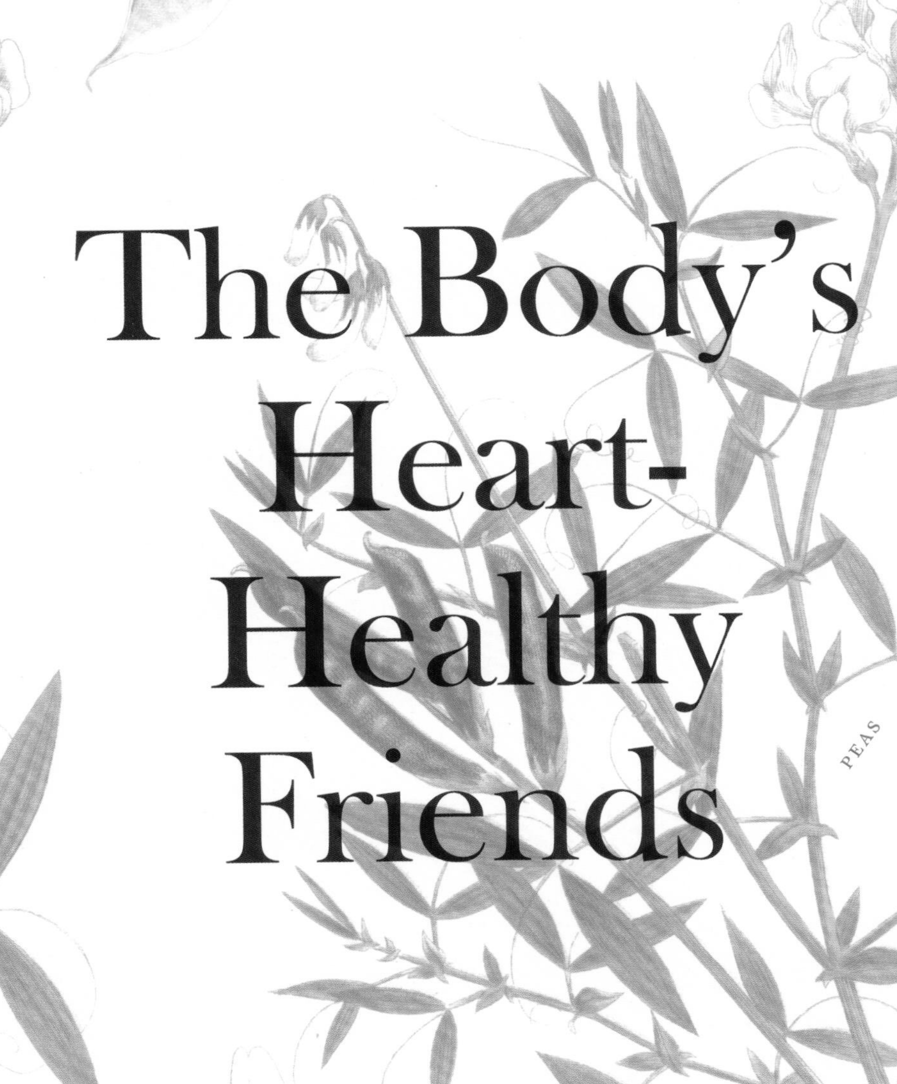

07

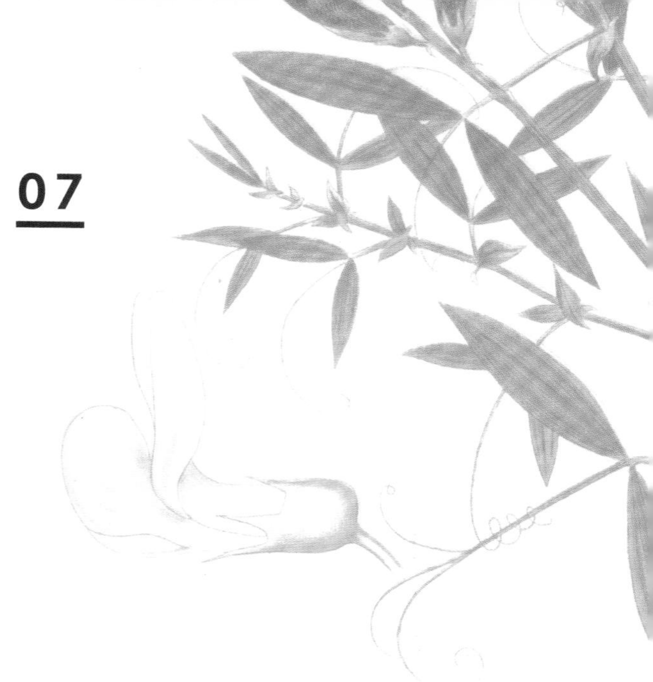

There are many truly heart-healthy friends for those of us who want to eat healthy. Not least the super gifted turmeric! Or the avocado, the kitchen magician. All the wholesome spices. The small glass of red wine and the hearty square of nearly pure chocolate. These are just fractions of all the favorite ingredients that are elevated in this chapter.

First an overview of our genes—our body's super piano—and also a look at eco-biological medicines, a suitable accompaniment to the genes' "instrumental."

THE HUMAN BODY has approximately 25,000 genes, 1,200 to 1,300 of which are involved in inflammation control. Add to this the 3 to 9 million genes that are our "in-house" bacteria, mainly in the intestines, that contribute heavily to controlling chronic inflammation in our body.

If we regard our genes as a super piano with 25,000 piano keys, the "inflammation symphony" produced depends wholly on how we treat/mistreat the keys. The more we hammer them with bad foods, stress, and lack of exercise, the worse the sound/effect. Some of us have more sensitive keys while others have more robust ones, that is, some of us will fall ill easier and others more seldom.

Probably all antioxidants possess a greater or lesser ability to "slow" the keys and are therefore able to adjust the harmful effects.

The Discovery of Turmeric

At the end of the last century, pharmaceutical companies realized what possibilities opened up if we could moderate chronic inflammation by dampening the effects of the involved genes. The hunt for inflammation inhibitors was on. These pharmaceuticals were given the collective name biological therapies. As it seemed impossible to inhibit all the 1,200–1,300 genes they focused on the especially powerful inflammation-provoking genes, like COX-2 (Prostaglandin-endoperoxide synthase 2).

But shock and horror! It turned out that most of the pharmaceuticals used against COX-2 were more or less toxic, causing death from cerebral hemorrhage and heart attack.

Many medical products had to be recalled and several pharmaceutical companies were forced to pay billions in damages. At one point in time there were many thousands of lawsuits for damages against pharmaceutical companies from individuals and families harmed.

Fortunately, plants and good bacteria possess the same function without the harmful effects. I call them ecobiologicals. The mission for these plant antioxidants (ecobiological supplements/ecobiologicals) used is instead to reach "as many genes as possible." Happily, this was a success! Certain spices have shown to affect most of the genes involved in inflammation—and turmeric exceeded expectations.

"The Queen of Plant Antioxidants: Turmeric"

A QUEEN AMONG PLANT ANTIOXIDANTS

Something amazing happened! Turmeric, an antioxidant picked straight from the plant kingdom, turned out to be a completely harmless inhibitor of the strongly inflammatory-backing genes COX-2, NF-kB (nuclear factor kappa-light-chain-enhancer of activated B cells) and many, many more. Turmeric can actually control nearly all the 1,200 to 1,300 most inflammatory-provoking genes, similar to what a high-class probiotic does. Turmeric and probiotics work excellently together.

Turmeric is a root, similar to ginger, but is smaller in size and a rich yellow. The Indian medical practice of Ayurveda has used turmeric for thousands of years to treat various internal and external medical conditions. Turmeric has been used just as long in different native medical practices.

Perhaps that is the reason why this spice is presented as something of a queen of antioxidants. It is possible there are other plant antioxidants that have similar effects—if they are explored.

I realized early on that turmeric had wide-ranging anti-inflammatory effects, something that Indians and other populations in Asia have known for a long time. Turmeric was initially used as a food preservative, especially in warmer climates. However, later on, it also was used to strengthen and preserve health. In contrast to biologicals, which are focused on silencing one gene at a time, turmeric silences the majority of active genes and in particular the most inflammatory-provoking. Both animal tests and human trials have shown strong clinical effects that I have written plenty about earlier on. The effects are achieved by use of different antioxidants but especially from the curcumenoid family. More than a hundred curcumenoids have been identified, and around twenty are in turmeric. Curcumin is the dominant antioxidant.

THE RESEARCH DELVES DEEPER

Clinical research into the effect of different substances is hugely expensive. Only pharmaceutical companies that may reap large benefits from their output have the resources to finance this. Money is usually not available for studies of things like turmeric and probiotics, and society hasn't shown a lot of interest in funding such work. This means that most research around these subjects, with a few exceptions, have centered on animal studies.

There are, however, many scientists researching the secrets of turmeric. In India, where they already have thousands of years of experience, more and more studies are being conducted.

According to the book *Herbal Medicine: Biomolecular and Clinical Aspects*, regular supplementation with turmeric gives considerable positive clinical effects both on animal and human subjects, notably where different cancers are present. It also protects and delays development of a variety of neurological diseases including both Alzheimer's disease and depression. It even protects against diabetes and various heart, blood vessel, and kidney diseases. What's more, turmeric also improves regeneration and healing of various joint and skeletal diseases.

These anti-infective effects may one day be expected to inhibit HIV (human immunodeficiency virus), influenza, and perhaps even the Ebola virus.

I have made repeated efforts to have these theories tried for Ebola—an inexpensive way that would fit African circumstances. However, I have received no response or understanding.

The University of Houston has a whole department devoted to research on turmeric. Illnesses and conditions they hope to be able to prevent and treat with turmeric/curcumin are, for example, allergies, cancer, diabetes, skin diseases, eye diseases, and skeletal diseases, as well as aging.

SO HOW DO YOU EAT TURMERIC?

It has been difficult to find fresh turmeric in the grocery stores until now. I've discovered, to my immense pleasure, more places now carry it.

Fresh turmeric is easy to work with. It can be diced finely and mixed directly into the salad. In India it is common to brush clean a few dozen turmeric roots (a week's worth) and store them in a mixture of half lemon juice and half water in a glass container. I've been told that people chew down two to three of these roots daily.

You will have to add a few ingredients if you take your turmeric in powder form. If not, it will be difficult for the body to take up enough of the turmeric. The uptake is facilitated by the addition of chili pepper and/or black pepper (as much as you can stand). This also increases the effect, as peppers in themselves are potent antioxidants/inflammation inhibitors.

The Avocado—One of the Miracle Fruits

Five of the newly introduced fruits now on sale in Sweden have received the collective label "the five miracle fruits." They are: avocado, coconut, longan fruit (from China), mango, and mangosteen.

Avocado was eaten in South America as early as 8,000 to 7,000 BCE. It reached North America at the beginning of the nineteenth century and has existed in Europe for only a few decades. The avocado truly is something of a health power station!

One of the avocado's virtues is that it is nearly sugar-free. One whole normal-sized avocado contains less than 1⁄60 of an ounce (½ g) of sugar (i.e., 3 calories or ⅕ of a sugar cube). Nevertheless, due to its rich fat content, it is still highly calorific. One avocado provides around 250 calories, which is the equivalent of an eighth (⅛) of the recommended daily calorie intake for an adult.

Another advantage of the avocado is that it is loaded with several appetite-suppressing and healthy plant fibers. It contains no fewer than ⅓ ounce (11 g) of fiber, nearly a third of the recommended daily requirement for an adult. The fiber composition is likened to the unripe green banana. The green banana used to be considered one of our very best fiber sources, and this fruit is worth a renaissance, in my humble opinion.

The avocado's protein content is also high at approximately ⅙ ounce (4 g)—in fact higher than we find in most other fruits.

What makes the avocado completely unique is its collection of fatty acids and its large amount of wholesome minerals, vitamins, and antioxidants. The necessary mineral potassium, as well as vitamin K, various B vitamins, vitamin C, and vitamin E are plentiful. The avocado is also rich in antioxidants such as alpha-carotene, beta-carotene, beta-cryptoxanthin, chrysanthemaxanthin, lutein, neochrome, neoxanthin, violaxanthin, and zeaxanthin. Physicians often recommend supplementing with lutein, because it has proven to counteract cataracts and protect the retinal macula.

The important amount of fat facilitates the bioavailability of these valuable substances.

COUNTERACTS FORMATION OF BLOOD CLOTS

Of all the good things we can say about the avocado, it is the fat content that makes it into a superfood.

Humans need fat in their diet—at least 10 percent, maybe even up to 30 percent of the daily calories. We've mentioned that our bodies cannot make certain fats, so we need to get them through our foods.

It is a definite advantage if foods are rich in short-chain fatty acids (SCFA) and medium-chain fatty acids (MCT), which are immediately delivered by the portal artery to be used by the liver. Coconut and palm oils are rich in MCT fats, and recently it was reported that even arugula lettuce contains MCT fats.

The avocado is certainly *not* rich in MCT fats but has another very important advantage in the fight against arteriosclerosis. It prevents "clotting" of platelets and the formation of blood clots, thus inhibiting the development of arteriosclerosis.

Some other plants which have shown themselves to possess the same unique properties, and are excellent tools as blood thinners, are turmeric and raw ginger. My wife and I willingly grate and eat turmeric or ginger, especially when we are going on longer plane journeys because of the high risk for developing blood clots. It was observed quite recently that some components of the avocado have the same properties.

"The avocado is next to unique—a health power-station."

Some physicians who prescribe blood thinners, like Warfarin and Trombyl, unfortunately dissuade their patients from consuming certain fruits and vegetables possessing similar properties. The list of substances that can delay coagulation is long, but as a rule the recommendations only catch a few of them. The preventive effect from Warfarin and Trombyl is in no way superior to the one provided with regular consumption of avocado and/or raw ginger.

I would prefer that we instead recommend regular use of plants like the avocado! They are not just more wholesome, they are also much cheaper than the commonly used drugs.

INFLAMMATION AND CANCER INHIBITING

Large parts of our population, especially the middle-aged and elderly, suffer from metabolic syndrome.

Clinical studies have shown that a daily intake of at least one avocado a day can lower the fat level and level of bad (LDL) cholesterol by an impressive 22 percent, and increase the good (HDL) cholesterol by at least 11 percent.

One of the avocado's benefits is an early feeling of satiety that, therefore, contributes to weight loss/lowered BMI (body mass index).

Studies have also shown that avocado has a strong inhibitory effect on cancer cells without being harmful to healthy cells. This has awakened hope that the avocado might be useful in so-called palliative cancer care. The strongest effect was observed on cancer cells from the esophagus, where two thirds of the effects are achieved with the cancer drug cisplatin (Platinol and others). Effects have also been found on colon and prostate cancer.

Additionally, the avocado "lubricates" joints and protects against osteoarthritis, the most common reason for joint replacements. Animal tests have shown significant histological and clinical improvement after treatment with a mixture of ingredients from avocado and soybeans.

REPLACES BUTTER AND CREAM

The avocado's large fat content has made it especially useful in daily meal preparations. In addition to eating it raw, it can also be used instead of cream in various dishes. Raw soups and smoothies become really creamy with the addition of avocado. The green banana can be used the same way (but it has nowhere near the same amount of fat and calories).

> "You can make gingerbread cookies using avocado instead of butter."

Enthusiasts claim that butter can often be replaced in a recipe with the same or double the amount of avocado. You can even make gingerbread cookies using avocado instead of butter.

In a modern household like ours where we eat a lot of raw plants, the avocado has become an invaluable part of the diet, just like the green banana. We always keep these fruits on hand in the freezer. If we get a visit from children, it is easy to quickly put together an avocado or banana ice cream by putting the fruits in a Vitamix together with raspberries or strawberries. The pieces of fruit are hardly suitable for snacking if they have been frozen, but they are excellent blended in smoothies and raw soups.

We are now waiting for the entrepreneur who shall take the idea and run with it and start to sell frozen green bananas and turmeric. This addition to food preparation would, according to our family, be as welcome as when the supermarket started stocking frozen green peas.

An Anti-Inflammatory Cocktail . . .

Many of the gut's favorite dishes aren't meant to be ladled in by the spoonful. Spices, for instance, do a whole lot of good even when it is just a pinch.

Nevertheless, in our kitchen we use many pinches. We use so many spices we have to buy them wholesale. We would be running out constantly if we didn't, and it would be too expensive to buy the ridiculously small tins the grocery stores offer.

A spice shot, an anti-inflammatory cocktail, isn't a bad idea if you want to profit from some selected items in the antioxidants league of champions (see list on p. 132).

The ability of different substances to keep at bay or strangle inflammation is quantified in an antioxidant index. The so-called ORAC (oxygen radical absorbance capacity) values are laboratory tested and must be interpreted with caution. The studied substances frequently don't give the hoped-for clinical effects, which may often depend on failed or too narrow uptake in the gut. However, it has been shown the uptake can be improved by the addition of fat; many antioxidants become fat-soluble after perfusion-stimulating steps, like the addition of chili pepper.

The list thus notes the plants that, so far, have shown the highest ORAC values. Cloves reign at the top. Cloves, an Indonesian spice, have been used for thousands of years in Asian medicine. It really ought to be called the world's most wholesome food. Cloves deserve to be used for so much more than sticking into oranges at Christmas for decorations and scent diffusers.

Cloves are closely followed by ground sumac bran, a lemon-tasting product which we use in smoothies and when baking bread at home. Durrah is our favorite for bread baking (not very handy yet, but we bake so seldom). We use mostly acai and other berries and cacao to blend with frozen avocado; or frozen, green, unripe banana for ice cream and desserts.

FOODS WITH HIGHEST ANTIOXIDANT CONTENT

ORAC µmol TE/31/2 OZ (100 G)

Food	ORAC
Cloves, ground	315,000
Sumac bran	312,400
Cinnamon from Ceylon	267,500
Durrah, raw, (bran)	240,000
Oregano, dried	201,000
Turmeric, ground	160,000
Acai berries, freeze dried	102,700
Sumak seeds	86,800
Cacao powder	81,000
Cumin	76,800
Parsley, dried	74,000
Durrah, red (thyme)	71,000
Basil, dried	61,000
Curry	48,500
Durrah, grain	45,400
Salvia, fresh	32,000

Source: U.S. Food and Drug Administration (FDA)

. . . AND ALL THE SECRETS IN MY BLOCKBUSTER SUPERMIX!

The most important ingredients in my introduced spice shot are turmeric, cloves, cinnamon from Ceylon, and chili pepper. The following explanation clarifies the mixture's health-bringing properties!

In this chapter I have already described in detail turmeric's unique character. This explains why it is such an important ingredient in my spice shot. The shot is rich in healthy minerals such as potassium, manganese, iron, selenium, and magnesium as well as various important vitamins such as vitamin A, beta-carotene, vitamin C, vitamin K, vitamin B6 (pyridoxine), and vitamin B (thiamine).

We have to add, the dominant curcumenoid and captain of the team is called *curcumin*. But the rest of the ingredients are just as important in their own way. It has been shown over the years that all are needed in various capacities to arrive at highest efficiency. The captain of the soccer can't win the match by making all the goals himself—he needs ten team players. The same is true in the world of curcumenoids.

Curcumin is sold in caplets, but don't buy them. Use the powder instead, or better still, fresh turmeric if you can find it.

Lately the clove may have inherited turmeric's crown as queen of antioxidants, because its ORAC value is the highest ever measured.

> "The clove has the highest ORAC value ever measured."

The clove is especially known for its rich oil content. It may contribute to the increased bioavailability of, for example, curcumenoids. The essential oil euginol (which is extracted from cloves) is attributed with wide-ranging health-enhancing properties. Euginol is an essential oil because it cannot be made by our body and has to be added from outside. Euginol has wide-ranging antiseptic and pain-relieving properties. It is therefore often used in dentistry as well as joint and muscle healthcare.

The clove is also attributed with the ability to speed up our gut's transit time of food (i.e., the gut motility) and to increase enzyme activity and digestion.

It also contains very large amounts of the chemical element manganese and is rich in many other things: vitamin K, iron, magnesium, and calcium, beta carotinoids, vitamin A, vitamin B6 (pyridoxine), thiamine (vitamin B-1), vitamin C, and riboflavin. The last components probably contributed to this spice's famous properties: anti-inflammatory, antiseptic (cleansing), anesthetic (to numb, elevate pain threshold), rubefacient (heating and soothing), and carminative (relief of bloating and flatulence).

In other lands, especially in Asia, this spice is used profusely, both for pleasure and health. It has a permanent place on the dining table in our home, together with a variety of peppers. Cloves go well with chicken (in a marinade or sauce), the same for fish or meat—combined gladly together with turmeric, chili pepper and ginger. It is also a nice seasoning for smoothies, soups, chutneys, and hot drinks such as tea and coffee.

The clove has been used very little in Western medicine. The nearest it has been used for medical purposes is the successful practice, at least in the United States, of using it as a temporary filling before proceeding to a root canal filling of teeth—precisely because of its unique ability to stave off inflammation and to act as a cleansing agent.

Cinnamon from Ceylon (*Cinnamomum verum*) is not to be confused with Cassia cinnamon (*Cinnamomum aromaticum*), Saigon cinnamon (*Cinnamomum loureroi*), or Botavia cinnamon (*Cinnamon burmannii*)—the harmful kinds of cinnamon sold in our stores. The difference in properties between these kinds and the healthy Ceylon cinnamon is considerable. The Ceylon cinnamon contains, among other things, nearly twenty times more antioxidants than the Saigon cinnamon.

Ceylon cinnamon contains considerably less coumarin than the Saigon and cassia cinnamon. I want to warn against using these two latter ones just because of this. Coumarin is a naturally occurring plant component that is toxic to the liver when consumed in larger amounts.

A regular intake of Ceylon cinnamon has shown to lower blood fats and body weight significantly and is therefore an effective tool for fighting metabolic syndrome and its consequences. Ceylon cinnamon is also known for its antidiabetic, antiseptic and anti-inflammatory properties.

For centuries, cinnamon has been one of the absolute standards on European tables. We've put it on our Swedish tables for decades. It is used by the teaspoonful each day in foods like muesli, smoothies, fruit, and other desserts; in chocolate and coffee; in frozen cubes for beverages, and in ice cream.

Like turmeric, cinnamon combined with other spices has shown itself able to lower quite dramatically the fat and glucose shock that is created after a meal, and at the same time it can significantly increase insulin sensitivity.

"Chili increases metabolism and is good for the digestion."

Big effects have been observed for blood fats. They actually decreased about a third. Another study, consisting of twenty-two subjects with metabolic syndrome and prediabetes, who were given a daily dose of cinnamon during several weeks, showed that the fasting blood sugar reduced 8 percent and the blood pressure 4 percent.

Other documented effects suggest that cinnamon can reduce the progress of neurodegenerative diseases such as Parkinson's disease, and contributes to better cardiovascular health. In fact, PubMed has 1,500 studies that highlight different effects of cinnamon—so please read an overview.

The chili pepper is chosen because of its unique characteristics to be able to appreciably increase the blood circulation through all the bodily organs. This increases the bioavailability of antioxidants and nutrition in the intestines, especially of the important turmeric/curcumenoids. Increased perfusion/hyperemia also contribute to a powerful ability to regenerate and heal, especially leg ulcers and similar conditions. In addition, an infusion of chili pepper results in less risk of amputation of organs like feet and legs, which unfortunately happens in cases of difficult-to-control diabetes.

Apart from all this, the chili pepper is attributed with characteristics such as being able to increase pain threshold. The ability to increase pain threshold and increase perfusion decreases the risk for blood clot formation and it counteracts "clogging" in organs, like nasal passages and the respiratory system. Reports also show positive effects for migraine headaches and joint pain.

As if this was not enough, chili pepper is said to increase metabolism and increase secretion of saliva, stomach acid, and other digestive fluids contributing to proper digestion. Increased perfusion also quite radically decreases problems from COPD (chronic obstructive pulmonary disease), chronic kidney disease (chronic dialysis), and chronic pancreatic insufficiency (diabetes, chronic pancreatitis).

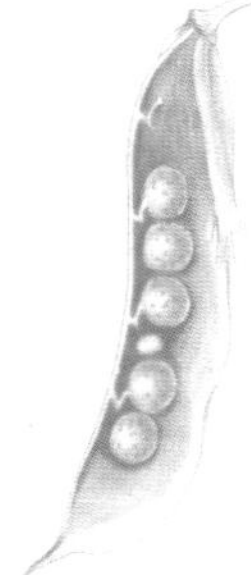

The Recipe—You Are Welcome!

First a word about dosage:

The common dose of turmeric in traditional folk medicine has been about a heaped tablespoon of turmeric powder. This can probably be reduced to a heaped teaspoon if mixed with other spices.

A suitable dosage of Ceylon cinnamon is a heaped teaspoon, but important clinical effects have been reported after a much smaller dose.

As for cloves, and especially chili pepper dosage, it is as much as you can tolerate. That means at least a big pinch (a quarter teaspoon).

This mixture can be consumed in many different ways, not just in a shot. You can sprinkle it on food. Why not try it on muesli and salads?

½ to 1 glass fruit juice—for example, pineapple, apple or similar
1 heaped tablespoon turmeric
Up to ¼ teaspoon cayenne pepper
½ to 1 teaspoon cumin, ground
1 dessert spoon (2½ teaspoons) Ceylon cinnamon
1 pinch (¼ teaspoon) cloves
½ to 1 tablespoon apple cider vinegar
1 teaspoon lemon juice

Mix all ingredients and drink twice daily. As an alternative, don't bother with the fruit juice. Just swallow the apple cider vinegar and sprinkle the spices on your food.

Smoothies and Green Beverages—Festive Everyday Mixes

A smoothie is a creamy or frothy beverage made from blended ingredients. Most of us make them from fruits and berries. Many add yogurt or some nondairy milk. Adding ice is good.

At home we make our smoothies with loads of frozen or fresh fruits, berries, and vegetables. As mentioned earlier, the avocado is a great replacement for any dairy ingredient in the recipe. Sometimes we prefer green beverages without any "milky" ingredients or too overt sweetness. Check out Marianne's super health drink, a green, rich-tasting beverage that gives just enough satiety.

The advantage with smoothies and green beverages is that they can hold so many raw and/or frozen nutrients all at once, not least, all the true super spices. Also all the truly nutritious plant pieces most people throw out—seeds, cores, leaves. You can pulverize them and add at will.

Imagine how much easier it would be to prepare and serve the children a tasty and wholesome meal if you just had frozen ingredients and a powerful kitchen blender at hand.

Pleasure—A Road to Health

Most, or perhaps all, of us have the need to take a break now and then; reward ourselves and celebrate that we've reached a goal or are partway there. Often it is something as simple as school or the workweek being over for a time. To have the opportunity to combine benefit with pleasure is truly fantastic!

The rest of this chapter will be all about stimulants. Healthy stimulants!

CHOCOLATE—THIS IS WHY IT MAKES YOU HAPPY

Chocolate actually belongs to the top group of food items that anybody can offer. It could be eaten in unending quantities if it wasn't for the calories. Admittedly, pure cacao has relatively few calories, only 230 calories/3½ ounces (100 g). However, a chocolate bar usually contains double the calories or more, because a lot of unwholesome ingredients like sugar and dairy products get mixed in.

To manufacture a "pure" chocolate bar they can use up to 86 percent pure cacao. If using a cacao percentage that is higher, it is difficult to make a chocolate bar that will hold together. So, either we are satisfied with "only" 86 percent or we can mix cacao ourselves with sweet-tasting berries that actually have relatively low sugar content. Some good examples are lime and lemon (0% sugar), cranberries, fresh apricots, cantaloupe (but no other type of melon), clementines and grapefruit (but no other citrus than these), pineapple, raspberries, strawberries, and red/white/blackcurrants.

Cacao contains two substances, anandamide and phenylethylamine (PEA), that are known for their ability to elevate the mood and counteract gloominess. Apart from containing a large amount of flavonoids, cacao is also known for its high content of magnesium and sulfur. Both are necessary elements for the body's repair, healing, and growth.

It has been observed that sulfur contributes to stronger nails and shinier hair. Remember, what you see on the exterior mirrors what is happening in the interior. Cacao also strongly counteracts illnesses associated with metabolic syndrome. Cacao is most known for making the blood vessel endothelium "smoother" and for counteracting arterosclerosis, heart attacks, and cerebral hemorrhages.

You can, however, overdose on cacao, and that's why adults are recommended to limit the daily intake to not more than 1½ ounces (40 g) pure cacao (approximately 6 heaped teaspoons).

TEA MAKES YOU HEALTHY

The science around tea is just as extensive as around wine. But while the general population's knowledge about wine is steadily growing, the knowledge about tea is decreasing dramatically. There are thousands of teas with different medicinal properties, each geared to its individual purpose: appetite suppressant (if you, for example, want to skip breakfast); stimulating and energy-giving when you are in need of this; and not least, the calming/soothing—for example, when the day is nearly over and you finish eating.

Heads up: Do not use tea bags! The bag, which usually contains the plastic compound epichlorohydrin, actually leaks plastic and plastic parts into the tea. Treat yourself to loose-leaf tea from a tea shop! At the same time treat yourself to a real gold filter, without any toxic plastic elements.

The quality of loose-leaf tea is absolutely superior to tea bags. Go ahead and empty a tea bag and compare the contents with loose-leaf tea. The bagged content is reminiscent of the waste at the bottom of each loose-leaf bag or, to sound slightly provocative, debris swept up off the floor. It will really surprise you.

Teas are rich in antioxidants—perhaps not quite as rich as the items I've mentioned earlier, but we compensate by drinking so much more tea.

"There are thousands of teas with medical effects."

My daily favorite tea is yerba maté, which comes from a South American Ilex plant (Ilex paraguariensis). The tea is easily found in tea stores, health food stores, and on the internet. Jesuit monks accompanied Columbus on his boats and drank the tea daily, especially as an appetite suppressant when they fasted. They brought other kinds of tea to Europe. After olive leaf tea, yerba maté is the richest in antioxidants that we know of to date. If you need to ease into the taste in the beginning, mix it with fruit teas.

Approximately 275 articles, research papers, and overviews on the health benefits of yerba maté tea are available in PubMed's archive. They report on the unique ability to act as a hunger suppressant, blood thinner, to increase blood flow through vital organs, achieve healthier blood glucose levels, prevent catastrophic vessel events, and to reduce body weight with consistent consumption.

Yerba maté's antioxidant content and its ability to "strangle" inflammation can be compared with green tea's and the well-known red wine's. It is a competition that yerba maté actually wins by a long shot.

Fermented teas like pu-erh tea are also highly recommended.

MODERATE AMOUNTS OF RED WINE—A HEALTH BOOSTER

Red wine possesses properties you won't find in any other wine. The great super antioxidants are extracted from the grape skins through a very specific manufacturing method. These are actually lactobacillus—not very different from the ones in the synbiotics I research daily—that separate the antioxidants from fibers in the skins and extract the goodness. The process is similar to the one going on in our gut.

Be alert though to disinformation and pure fraud around wine! As we know, this exists in all industries, from tobacco to pharmaceuticals, and also today in the food industry. However, the suspicion is that the wine industry leads the way in this.

Murky interests protect this industry that is also greatly cherished by, among others, the EU (European Union). For example, there are no regulations for declaring content and additives. It seems to me that no other industry is in as much need of oversight and legal regulations as wine producers. Also be aware that grapes are one of the most-sprayed fruit crops. The pesticides unfortunately end up in the wine. Add to this, there are around fifty additives the producers work with. The organic wines are not without blame either. EU has now decided to take vigorous action against all this. Nevertheless, as long as the situation is unsolved, I only buy organic wines and organic brut/champagne.

It has to be admitted though that today's enologists are very good at making even tasty synthetic wines, something they would like to reap the benefit from. I've been told in certain countries the legislation only demands a bottle contains as little as one real grape for the contents to be allowed to be marketed as wine. This does not apply to countries with thousand-year-old traditions of winemaking. There the industries' own code of ethics demands that the wines sold are the real thing.

One glass of red wine contains the same amount of antioxidants as three glasses of natural grape juice, that is, from the same, but unfermented, grape.

Antioxidant content reveals how the wine was manufactured but sadly, this can be falsified too, by addition of antioxidants to "synthetic" wines.

Professor Leroy Creasy at Cornell University has spent his working life researching wine and antioxidants and is today one of the world's leading experts in the field. He says that pinot noir constantly holds the highest levels of the super antioxidant resveratrol, which is also found in large amounts in fresh raw peanuts. Cabernet, Syrah, and merlots contain most of a partly different group of antioxidants. Precisely, that other group has shown itself to reduce inflammation in the body, exert blood-thinning effect, and therefore reduce blood-clotting risk and generally benefit cardiovascular health. The general rule, on the whole, is that the darker, the more rustic, and drier the wine is, the more antioxidants it contains. Creasy's main advice is to buy your wine from the small wineries that have, if possible, their vineyards in the vicinity.

When I can choose myself, I'll drink wines from Northern Italy, Southern France, and Corsica. My personal summary: Preferably choose organic wines or organic sparkling wines. If that's not possible, go for pinot noir, Syrah, or merlot—preferably from a vineyard within a fifteen-mile radius of Monaco.

A group of English researchers decided to investigate, on the one hand, the ability to "snuff out inflammation," and, on the other, the existence of super-antioxidants in various red wines.

ORAC values are, after all, only a fiftieth of the values for cloves, turmeric, and cinnamon.

So, gladly raise a glass! But avoid hard liquor. Don't forget that wine contains alcohol, which is just as harmful as sugar, nor its possible social consequences. Drink at most one bottle of wine a week, and then only red wine. I drink much less and usually only at weekends or festive occasions.

The French for "cheers" is "*a votre santé!*" (To your health!) That's just what you will get with sensibly chosen pleasures.

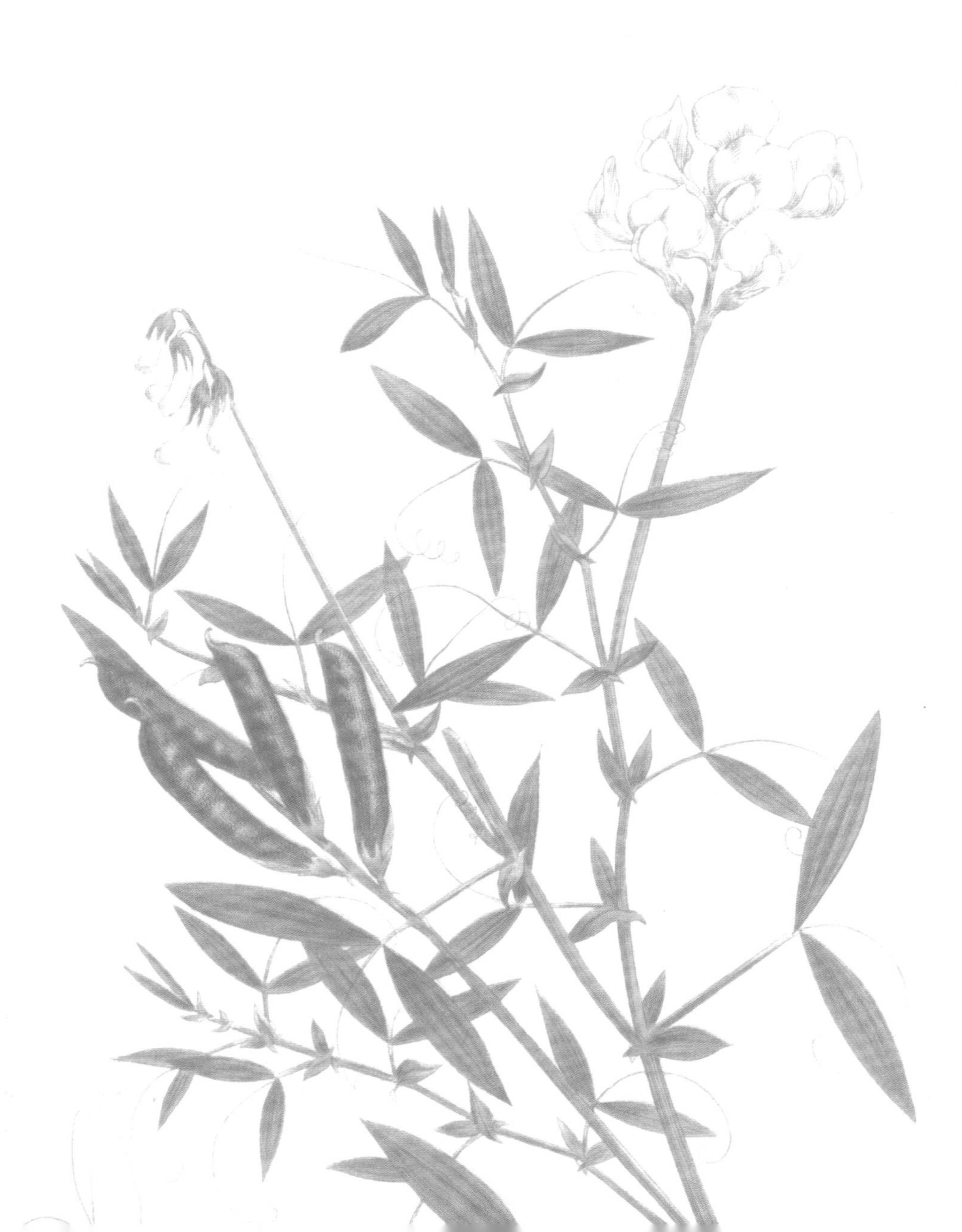

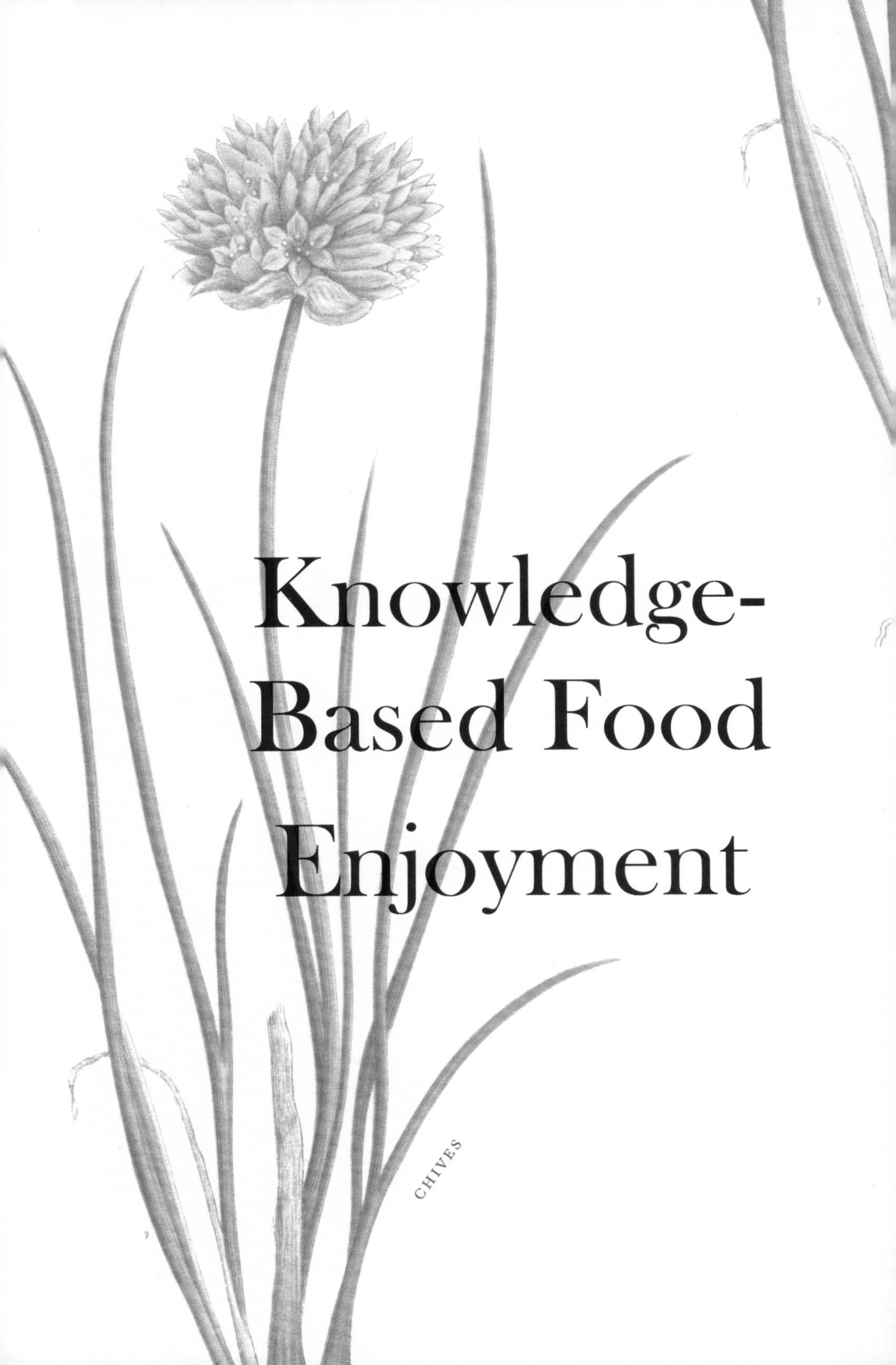

Knowledge-Based Food Enjoyment

08

What do you really learn by checking out the store shelves or reading the text on packaging when you're shopping for food? Not much!

In this chapter I want to give you useful basic knowledge about various food ingredients and everyday dealing with them. You will also get tips on how to avoid ruining their vital nutrients. Trust me: Food is so much tastier when you know that it is also good for your body and irreplaceable digestive system. Food enjoyment increases with knowledge!

MARIANNE AND I carry a cheat sheet in our wallets where it's written:

> avocado, pineapple, cabbage, onion, asparagus, mango, papaya, kiwi, eggplant, grapefruit, cantaloupe, cauliflower, sweet potatoes

This is a list of vegetables we eat with pleasure. They are welcome in our kitchen because of a truly exceptional reason. These vegetables have shown to contain so little spray residue (from pesticides) they don't even have to be bought as organics. Now that's happy news!

A Guide to the Vegetable Jungle

In fact, we carry a second cheat sheet. On it is the Dirty Twelve, also known as the Dirty Dozen. These fruits and vegetables, and probably more, should only be consumed if you can find them organically grown because they retain a lot of pesticide residue. (I'm not totally certain that the label "organic" isn't exaggerated sometimes . . . I still need to be convinced.)

Sadly, several of our favorites that are known for their great nutritional value are on The Dirty Dozen list.

> apples, strawberries, grapes (wine), celery, peaches and nectarines, spinach, red and green bell peppers, cucumbers, cherry tomatoes, sugar peas, and potatoes

We make exceptions and still buy some of them. But do remember to only buy organically grown! The alternative is to avoid them totally and look for other safer fruits and vegetables. Perhaps a boycott of pesticide-sprayed produce could be effective?

THE NUTRITIONISTS' RECOMMENDATION

Nutritionists have tried to present a list of fruit and vegetables to replace the Dirty Dozen. Here's the third cheat sheet!

The list really needs to be longer because the amount of "hidden" produce is very large. Nevertheless, what you see here is the one we start from. I suspect it is going to be revised incrementally as we get more information. This is, of course, already very useful today!

"DIRTY DOZEN"	CAN BE REPLACED BY THESE OTHER GOOD-FOR-YOU ITEMS:
STRAWBERRIES	Blackberries, raspberries, blueberries, kiwi, orange, cantaloupe
SPINACH, LETTUCE, NECTARINES	Broccoli, Brussels sprouts, asparagus, parsley, watermelon, raspberries, redcurrants, romaine (Cos) lettuce
APPLES	Cantaloupe, watermelon, tangerine, grapefruit
GRAPES & WINES	Banana, kiwi, watermelon, tangerine, mango, organic wines
PEACHES	Cantaloupe, tangerine, grapefruit
CHERRIES	Grapefruit, wild blueberries, tangerine, raspberries, cantaloupe
CELERY	Orange, banana, kiwi, watermelon, tangerine, mango
POTATO, SQUASH	Sweet potatoes, carrots
GREEN BELL PEPPER	Green peas, broccoli, Romaine (Cos) lettuce
RED BELL PEPPER	Carrots, broccoli, Brussels sprouts, tomatoes, asparagus

Source: The Environmental Working Group

Eat lots of plant foods—at least 1¾ pounds (800 g) to 2¼ pounds (1 kg) a day. Eat the foods as fresh and raw as possible. Defrosted frozen is also good. Look for foods that are particularly rich in antioxidants, plant fiber, and plant protein. Use gluten-free grains like amaranth, durrah (sorghum), teff, quinoa, seeds, peas, beans, lentils, almonds, and nuts. Soak dried foods in water for 12 to 24 hours before eating them.

FROM MY TWELVE COMMANDMENTS FOR OPTIMAL HEALTH, P. 74

CHOOSE ONLY THE BEST!

Celery, bell peppers, spinach, and kale are among our absolute favorite vegetables. As we really don't want to do without them (even if they belong to the Dirty Dozen), we only buy organically grown. For convenience sake, we like to have plenty of frozen organically grown vegetables at hand. Both spinach and kale keep their nutritional value superbly when frozen. The food industry doesn't seem to have caught on quite yet. How often do we find organic produce in the freezer section?

We're especially pleased that broccoli passes the pesticide-free test. This means more broccoli on our plates in the future. We also note, with pleasure, that this green list promotes parsley (don't just sprinkle it as decoration on the plate, eat it as salad), thyme, and chard (my father called it "poor man's asparagus").

Another positive point is that cantaloupe is highlighted in this context. This is the only kind of melon we eat regularly, as it has much less fructose in comparison with other melons like watermelon. Cantaloupe's sugar content is equal to that of raspberries, and is much lower than that of, for example, apples and pears.

FLASH FREEZING IS A SUCCESS

Vegetables quickly lose a lot of their freshness and antioxidant content right after being harvested. Earlier we had the example of the head of lettuce that loses half of its antioxidants half an hour after it is separated from its roots.

Frozen peas, which are extremely nutritious, are nowadays flash frozen at harvesting—a real success! This method ought to be used for many more kinds of vegetables.

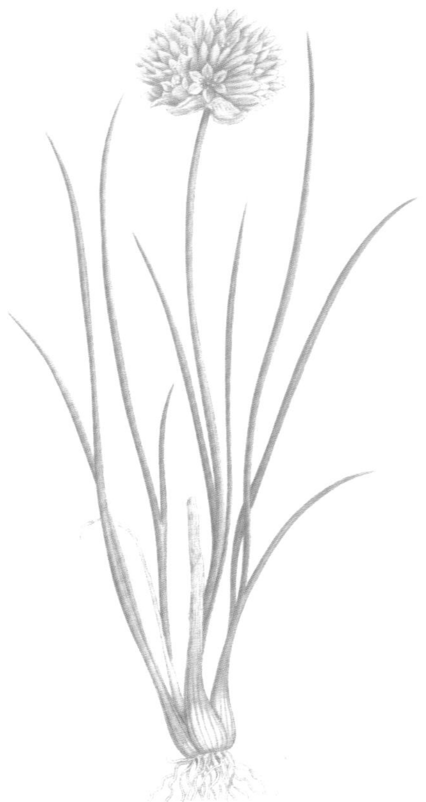

Overall, freezing seems to preserve both nutritional value and antioxidant amount relatively well (with a few exceptions). Rushed and stressed adults can, with a clear conscience, use various handy frozen vegetables that are often cheaper than fresh produce.

Perhaps one day we will flash-freeze sugar beet greens in the field to sell for human consumption, while the beet goes to feed the cows.

One day may arrive when other legumes aren't routinely dried before becoming human food. Instead, they'll be flash frozen in the fields before being shipped off to the grocery stores. Let's hope!

I personally lobby frozen food producers to start freezing and marketing the miraculous mung bean—an ingredient we often use in our salads as an alternative to quinoa.

SHOP FRESH, RAW, AND FROZEN

We touched on this earlier: It is the food manufacturers (and also yourself) who destroy precious and nutritious fiber and antioxidants through unnecessary heating and cooking.

> "Unripe plants are extremely rich in both fiber and antioxidants."

Apart from this, valuable fibers are transformed into sugar when fruits such as bananas, apples, and pears ripen. To eat raw and fresh is therefore an important principle for good health. This is a good reason to buy, as an alternative, many fruits and vegetables frozen. Hopefully they are flash frozen at harvest time.

Remember that many unripe plants are very rich in both fibers and antioxidants. When plant fibers ripen, they are converted into simple sugars. The unripe banana is a typical example of a fruit enormously rich in fiber, especially pectin, but when ripe it turns mostly into sugar and calories.

We never buy yellow (we call them "half putrid") bananas because of this knowledge. We strike when they are green and difficult to peel and stick to the palate when we eat them. We buy plenty when they are available and freeze them unpeeled for later use. We did the same earlier on with avocados, but we don't have to do this any longer as we can buy them already frozen. We just spoon out the content and mix with various other fruits when we want to make ice cream or some other dessert.

Even the potato is rich in pectin. This pectin unfortunately turns into sugar when the potato is cooked, but then converts back to fiber once the potato cools down. Our ancestors consumed plant matter long before it was ripe, and even wild apes do this. My understanding is we ought to develop a technique to be able to harvest plants like seeds and grains perhaps two to three weeks earlier than we traditionally do. Of course, that requires completely different harvest equipment than what we presently have available.

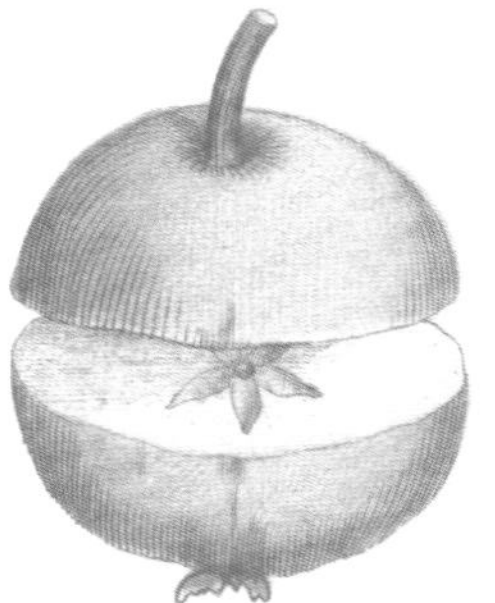

Aim to consume fresh or freshly frozen fruit and vegetables and choose items with a low glycemic index. Use lots of inflammation-reducing spices: ground cloves, turmeric, and different kinds of peppers. Like chili pepper? Go for it! Also drink inflammation-inhibiting teas like pu-erh and yerba maté. Eat whole olives but avoid the oil. Supplement year-round with vitamin D, omega-3, turmeric, and probiotics/synbiotics—the four cornerstones of an anti-inflammatory regime. Go ahead and add iodine in the form of potassium chloride or kelp.

FROM MY TWELVE COMMANDMENTS FOR OPTIMAL HEALTH, P. 74

DIVERSITY, LUKEWARM AND RAW

A tip from those of us who let vegetables dominate the meal:

Go for diversity in your intake of slow carbohydrates! Place many varieties on the plate. Put perhaps only one potato on the daily lunch or dinner plate and add a broccoli floret, some Brussels sprouts, cauliflower, and one or two other root vegetables such as carrot, parsnip, or celeriac.

If you want to warm the vegetables, as I mentioned before, do it gently—steam them rather than boiling them in water. All your various vegetables can be steamed together in the same saucepan (where they will stay put instead of tumbling around). This is an excellent method to use for the fish you might choose to complete the meal.

> "Go for diversity in your intake of slow carbohydrates!"

Remember that heated potatoes and root vegetables get back most of their wholesomeness if you let them cool down before eating. It's therefore easy to simplify the food preparation by, for instance, cooking potatoes to last several days. Perhaps you'll eat them warm the first day and then cold the following days.

I personally prefer cold potatoes, as I think they are tastier than warm ones. Hand on heart, isn't that the charm with raiding the refrigerator—the servings of cooled-down leftovers?

New Grain Varieties, Thank You!

It's time to discover newer and more wholesome grain varieties, which fortunately, many have already understood. For me, the focus can be directed toward breakfast cereals and porridge. This is in contrast to breads, as bread baking demands high temperatures that are far too harmful.

For decades I excluded the useless refined wheat flour in my own kitchen. This flour contains mostly empty calories. Also excluded in our household are the gluten-bloated and overrefined rye, wheat, and barley grains. Oats are still OK—they're actually really good! It's important to know the ratio between bran and flour—the nutrients are concentrated mostly in the bran.

Even corn and common millet are banned in Marianne's and my kitchen nowadays. We use quinoa, buckwheat, and more and more of the newcomer durrah/sorghum, also called Indian millet. However, we do see degenerative traces from plant breeding even among the new products. It is especially obvious in quinoa, which has gotten a more floury texture over the years.

Our ancestors' grain is arriving in leaps and bounds—the ADT-grouping of amaranth, durrah (Indian millet), and teff—immense power! We, the humans, homo sapiens, originate from Africa and now—a few thousand years later—our ancient grains arrive in Europe.

Dear plant breeders, we know that you have already got these grains in your clutches. But we beg you: for our health's sake, leave them be!

Apart from the fact that grains like the ADT group are less bred, they also have decidedly lower calorie content and a much higher content of wholesome vitamins and minerals than the conventional grains. This is especially true for durrah, Indian millet/sorghum, which is also richer in antioxidants (see table) when compared with fruits and vegetables. Keep an eye out for these plants and use them in your daily meals!

DURRAH—AN OLD-WORLD SUPERSTAR AMONG GRAINS

Durrah (sorghum/Indian/great millet, jowari, milo) has superior health-promoting properties compared to traditional grains. More particularly, it is the world's best and most nutritious grain. It is shameful that it is hardly used in Europe.

Durrah is not the easiest grain for baking bread, but it is possible! It can also be used to make muesli, in food preparation, to make plant milk and in lots of other ways.

As is evidenced by the following table, durrah contains significantly more antioxidants than other great things we eat with pleasure: blueberries, strawberries, plums, broccoli, carrots, and onions.

ANTIOXIDANT ACTIVITY IN DURRAH COMPARED TO OTHER FOODS' ORAC

(µmol TE/3½ OZ (100 G), DRY WEIGHT)

Tannin durrah (grain)	45,400
Tannin durrah (bran)	240,000
Black durrah (grain)	21,900
Black durrah (bran)	100,800
Red durrah (grain)	14,000
Red durrah (bran)	71,000
White durrah (grain)	2,200
White durrah (bran)	6,400
Blueberries	9,600
Strawberries	4,300
Plums	8,050
Apple, Red Delicious	4,275
Orange	2,100
Broccoli	3,080
Carrot	700
Red onion	1,520
Green bell pepper	935
Radishes	1,750
Potatoes	1,680

The Worst of the Worst Among Flours: Corn and Millet

Among all grains and ingredients used to make flour, perhaps it is corn that the plant breeders have done the most damage to. It is also corn that is most often destroyed by genetic modification.

Once upon a time, the corncob was very small in size but contained more of many different nutritional values than today's overbred corn does. It was, as usual, greed and the demand for increased crop yield that pushed the development of the product we have today. Today's corn is not fit for human consumption, in my honest opinion. I would prefer not to see it as animal feed, either—mainly because of the environmental issues. Each year large areas of rain forest are devastated to satisfy the need for corn for animal feed, primarily for meat and milk production.

"Today's corn is not fit for human consumption, in my honest opinion."

The global production of corn is already vast. It is estimated that it will continue to increase rapidly also in the future—which means increasingly serious environmental damage. A dramatic reduction in the demand for meat and dairy products is really the only thing that can stop this development.

Corn flour is, just like rice flour, junk flour that none of us need. These flours, like other products from these plants, all have unacceptably high GI values.

Millet is now in the bull's-eye as a grain to be avoided. This was unexpected, and enormously disappointing to me because many like me have always seen millet as wholesome.

There are several reasons why millet is shown to be dubious: The GI is comparatively high: 101. It contains a large amount of saponins that are known to increase leaky gut. Millet is also rich in phytic acid/phytate, a substance that binds to minerals such as iron, calcium, zinc, and magnesium. This impairs the body's ability to absorb these minerals.

In addition, millet also contains very little iodine, an essential trace element.

CORN—THE WORST OF THE WORST

Corn is unusually calorific and often it is enhanced by large amounts of sugar. A study of the calorific content of popcorn sold in London's movie theaters showed the cones/bags contained more than 1000 calories—a calorific content equal to at least half of the recommended daily intake for a fifteen-year-old.

The sugar usually added to popcorn doesn't just increase the calorie content; it also contributes to the corn's ability to induce elevated inflammation in the body. Corn is, unfortunately, no longer just eaten by children and adults during the occasional movie visit. It is eaten quite regularly when relaxing on the couch in front of the television at home. In many families this is an appreciated part of what Swedes call "Friday Cosy."

However, it is neither the calorie content nor the sugar that makes corn "the worst of the worst." There are far too many competitors for that one. What makes corn especially problematic is its content of the gluten and casein-similar proteotoxic zein. Zein is used in the manufacturing of various plastic products used for leakproofing paper drinking cups, sealing fabrics, for buttons, and just like the gluten in the past—as glue.

Zein in foods has had catastrophic influence on activation of neurotransmitters, especially serotonin and melatonin as well as adrenaline and dopamine—all with the common name monoaminer.

I'm convinced that we all will feel so much better if we abstain from corn, corn products, and probably also millet. This is important for sufferers of neuropsychiatric illnesses, perhaps especially everybody diagnosed with an "acronym diagnosis." Amphetamine, which is commonly used in treatment of ADHD, has a molecular structure that is very similar to tryptophan—perhaps it works because it acts as a tryptophan substitute.

Who Wants to Harm Their Great-Grandchild?

How corn is shown the door in my home is perhaps an unusually explicit explanation how healthy eating needs knowledge; continuously updated knowledge. Also how knowledge creates its demands on how you eat.

I have long known that corn is sweet and ruined through breeding. But now I have to add the new findings about the composition of corn to my already existing knowledge. Your attitudes change in step with what you learn.

If someone had said to me when my grandchildren were small, "oh come on Stig, give the children some popcorn, as you're going to the movies," I probably would have said OK. However, today, when I know that the zein in corn can break down the monoamines—yet, recognizing how monoamines are lacking in the brain with illnesses like ADHD and depression—how on earth can I give popcorn to a loved great-grandchild?

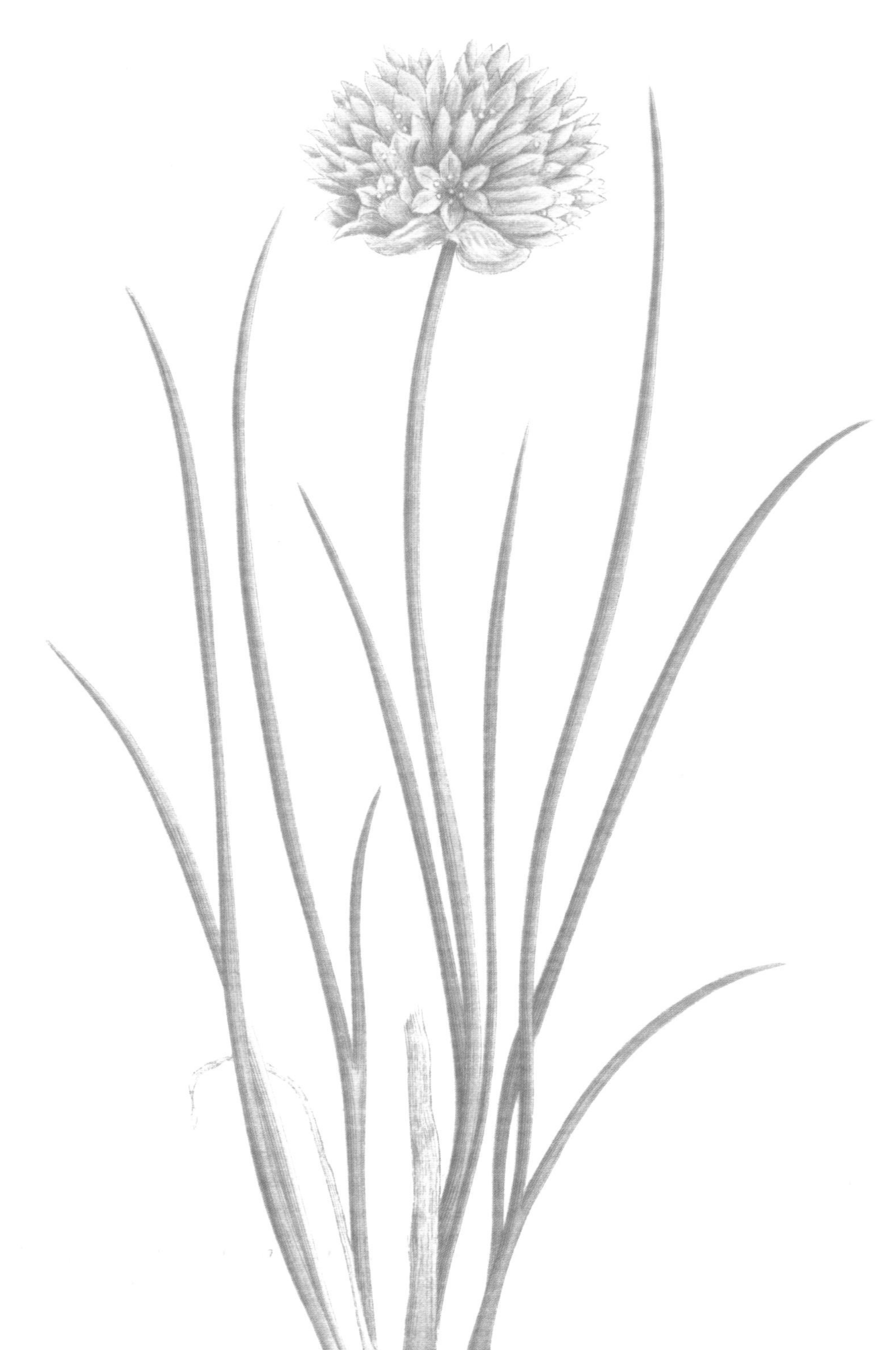

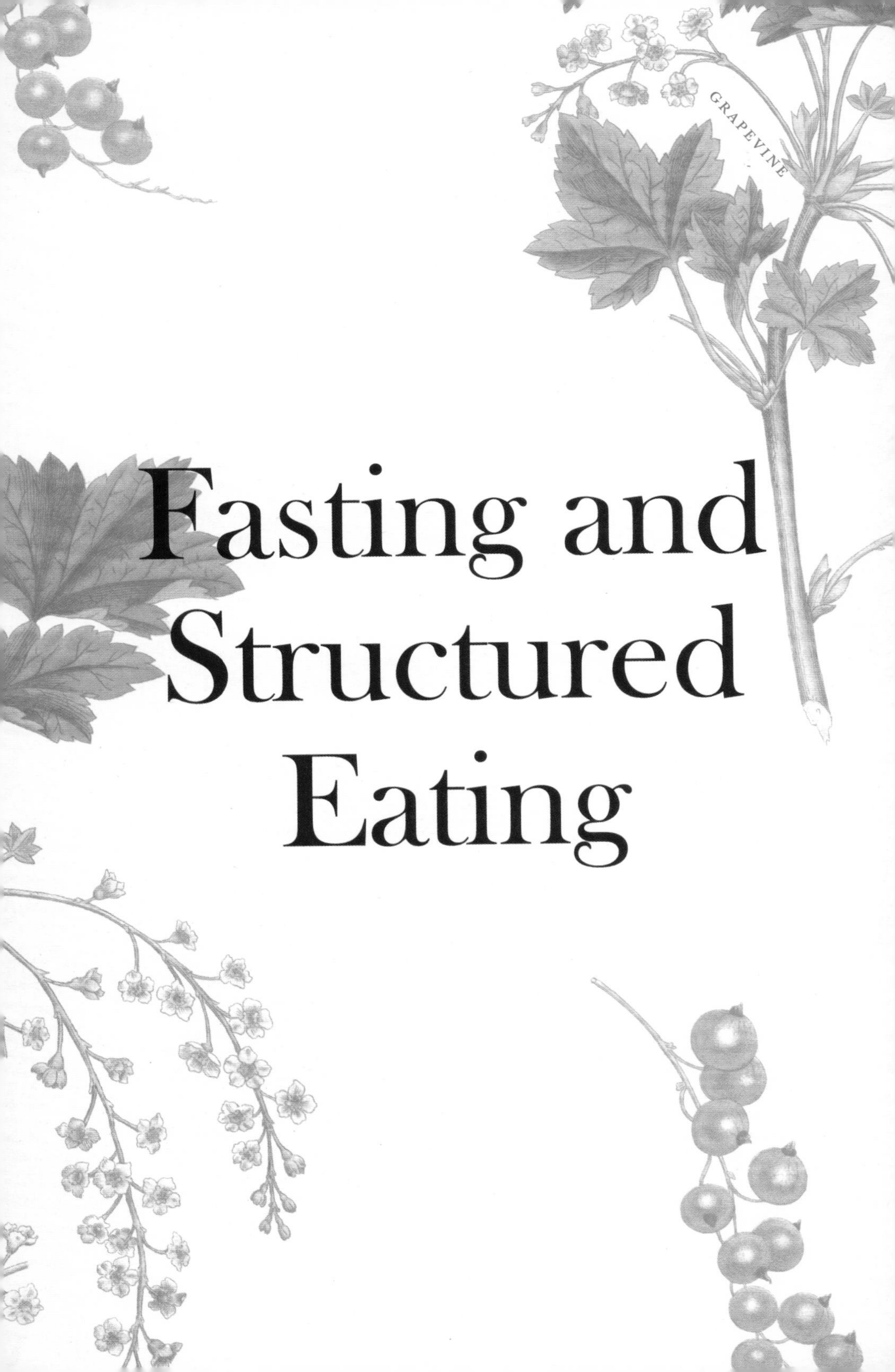

Fasting and Structured Eating

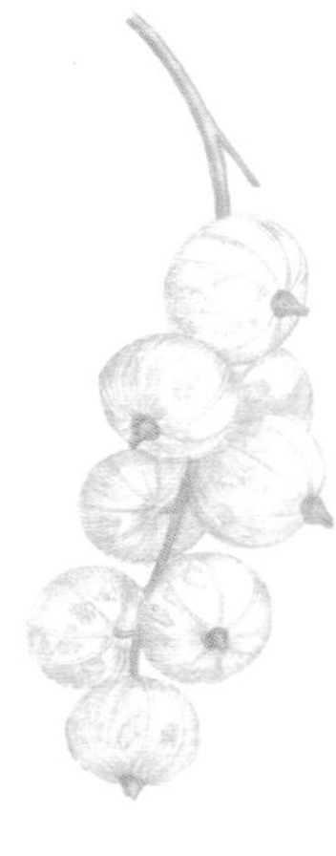

09

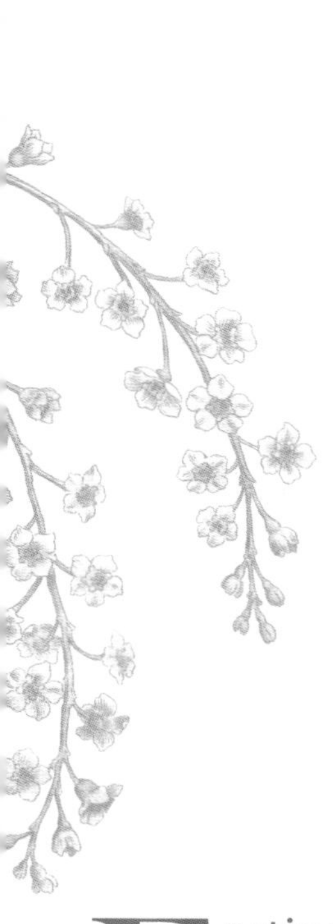

Fasting for short periods or for a larger part of the day—these are ideas and needs that humans have practiced as far back as they can trace ancestry.

In our days, when meals have become considerably less ritualized than in our grandparents' time, new needs for structured meals have arisen. There might be various reasons for this: spirituality and tradition, rest and cleansing, recuperation or weight loss.

Here is something about the meaning, methods and the new findings—from the perspective of the Anti-Inflammatory Diet!

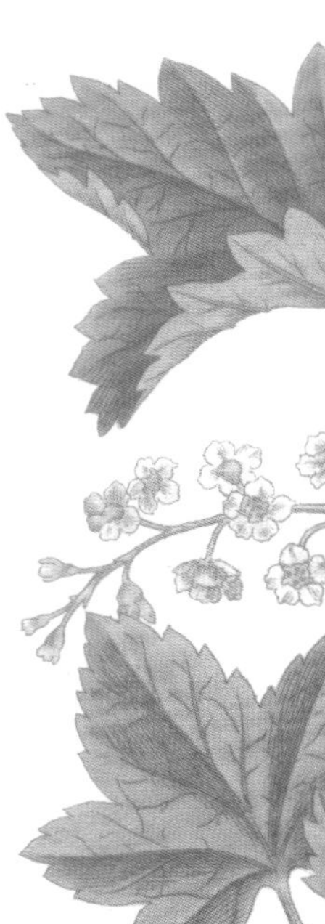

FASTING IS NOT a recent phenomenon. The need, both spiritual and health-related, to fast every now and then was born early among humans. As early as 2000 to 3000 BCE, Moses fasted for forty days in the desert.

Our ancestors lived like hunters and gatherers for millions of years. They ate what the season gave. As long as they stayed in Africa, food was usually abundant and varied. The diet consisted mostly of flowers, leaves, and roots.

Our ancestors' diet might give the impression of being a permanent fasting cure. Translated to modern diet habits it approached the 80/10/10 method. Their consumption of fish and meat varied a lot, but it was often rather limited.

"Fasting's benefits came to be regarded as important parts of life."

When humans started to "burn" food its quality was impaired and no longer as healthy. It wasn't until agriculture entered the picture, however, that food quality deteriorated more drastically.

Food became more available and, therefore, easier to abuse; choices definitely became more narrow.

Opportunity for overeating increased noticeably and the disadvantages were evident. Gluttony was regarded as a deadly sin; in the Old Testament moderation is held up as a virtue. Eating was eventually relegated to only twice a day. Some people follow this even today. Fasting's benefits came to be regarded as important parts of life and in the religious calendar.

Fasting Cultures in Our Days

Fasting still exists as a practice and in all religions. The most well-known is Ramadan, the Muslims' month of fasting. Some might oppose the way Ramadan is sometimes performed, but everybody ought to respect the important psychological and physical improvements that are reported during and after a completed Ramadan.

Traditional fasting by cultures can still be studied in some distant parts of the globe like Abkhazia in Georgia by the Black Sea, Vilcabamba in Ecuador, and in the Hunza region of northern Pakistan. The inhabitants there don't practice periods of fasting; a better explanation is that they actually practice fasting daily. They seldom eat processed foods, and the communities that consume dairy products (mostly Abkhazians) drink their milk unpasteurized and fermented. The Vilcacambians and Hunza inhabitants are virtually vegans.

These ethnic groups live on an average of 1,700 to 1,800 calories a day, even though they work long days in the fields. (Compare this with what the Nordic Nutritional Recommendations suggests: 1,800 to 2,400 calories for women, and 2,300 to 3,000 calories for men, even if many consume much more.) Inhabitants in the ethnic areas are seldom ill, and surprisingly large groups of people live to be more than a hundred. Okinawa in Japan was long known as the place on earth where people were healthiest and had the longest life span. However, after the Americans built military bases on Okinawa after World War II's end, the inhabitants partly adopted a lifestyle that changed their health and life span status radically. Today, the island's health status is one of the worst of Japan's fifty different regions.

New Ideas about Structured Eating

When the gorillas in the Cleveland Zoo became very obese on a Western diet, they were put on a meal plan consisting of only romaine lettuce, frisée lettuce, alfalfa hay, tree branches, beans, flaxseed, and a banana dipped in multivitamins. They lost 66 lbs. (30 kg) in about one year, and they now weigh the same as gorillas in the wild.

Animal studies show the importance of structured eating. Two groups of mice in one study were given the same amount of calories. However, one group could feed at will, while the other group could only eat for less than half the day (see diagram). The animals that were allowed to feed freely became fatter and fatter, and also sicker and sicker. Especially their livers suffered, as they were never given a rest. The mice developed problems with glucose (glucose intolerance increased) and their muscle function (motor coordination). The satiety hormone leptin's ability was blunted (leptin resistance). The mice in the group with a daily fasting period became slimmer and slimmer and healthier and healthier, despite consuming the same amount of calories.

A few years ago, the BBC asked nine individuals to, during two weeks, eat very similar foods to what the ancient hunter/gatherers would have eaten. It was mainly raw foods and very little fat. The nine mostly ate broccoli, carrots, melons, figs, nuts, plums, radishes, bananas, strawberries, cabbage, tomato, garden cress, apricots, and mangoes—with some fish now and then. The participants, who on average lost eleven pounds (5 kg), didn't feel that they lost any energy and they were in good spirits during most of the time. Just two weeks of eating an "ancestral" diet brought plenty of health benefits. Many blood values improved markedly, and cholesterol, for example, decreased 23 percent.

Fasting, a Recuperation

Generally, fasting has become more common today in nondenominational settings in the West, mostly as a way to cleanse the body of toxins. Our health research shows an ever-growing interest for the lifestyle that most resembles our ancestors' lifestyle.

Limiting intake of food, called calorie restriction (CR)—where you permanently or periodically eat only about 2/3 of the amount you really would like—has shown itself to have important effects on health. Animal experiments show a doubling of life span, significantly lowered illness, and an important delay in onset of chronic illnesses.

DAILY FASTING PREVENTS OBESITY AND PROMOTES BETTER HEALTH

A mice study showed that the group that restricted their eating to less than half the day improved their health in many ways.

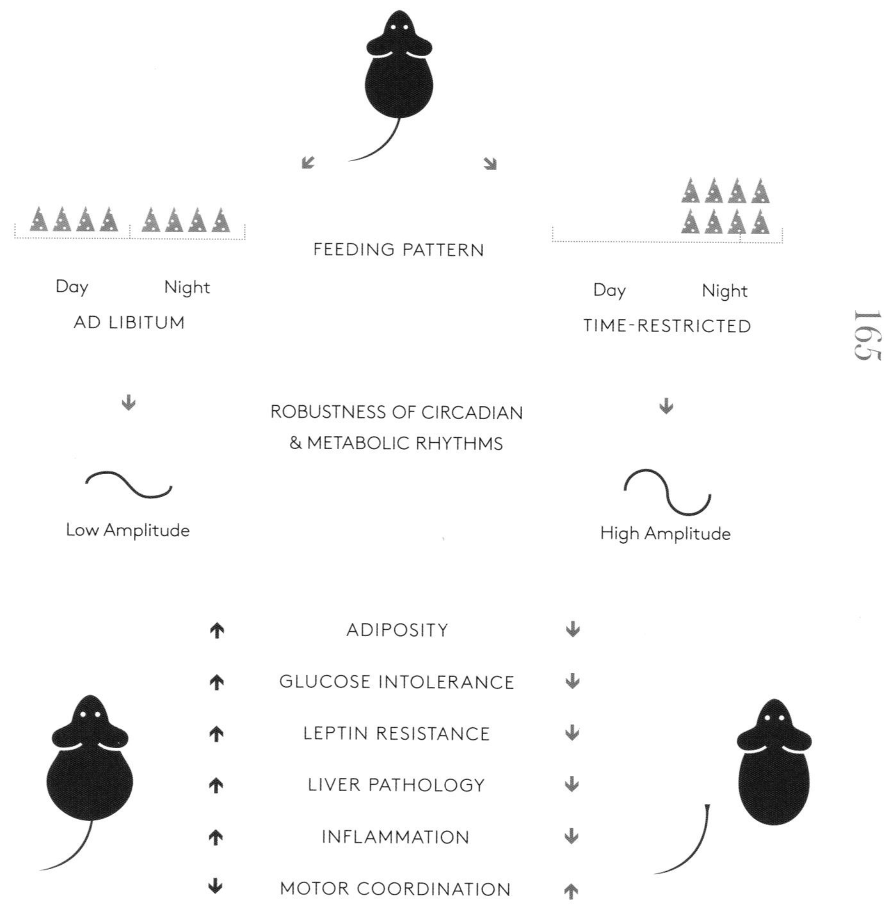

Source: Hatori, M. et al.

FOOD CONSUMPTION DURING TIME-RESTRICTED FEEDING VERSUS AD LIBITUM PER 24 HOURS

Further studies showed how mice with different starting points responded to different calorie amounts, and different time schedules, both for a twenty-four-hour period and for the week. Note that even the lower calorie intake during free feeding led to morbid obesity in the first example.

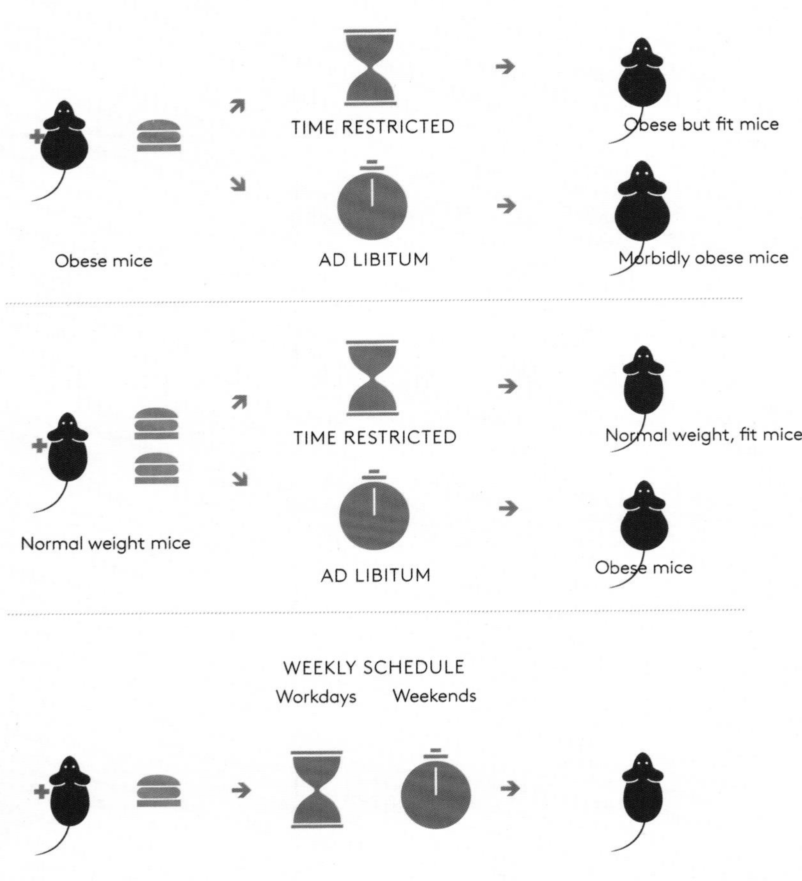

Source: Chaix, A. et al

Even if human studies haven't yet become as extensive as we wish, renowned researchers report important progress when applying CR also to humans. For example, there is reduced risk of getting cancer, diabetes, or cardiovascular disease. In American studies, overweight individuals lost 1 percent of body weight per week, which actually is as good a result as seen after bariatric surgery. They also avoided side effects and disadvantages to the digestive system commonly experienced after surgery.

"A daily structured fasting period has shown to confer several benefits. It gives our organs the time to rest and recuperate."

To achieve the effect of CR, it looks like it is vital to restrict protein intake; especially the amino acid methionine, which is plentiful in animal products.

A daily structured fasting period has shown to confer several benefits. It gives our organs the time to rest and recuperate—which results in this:

- whole body fat accumulation is greatly reduced, especially in the circulatory system and liver
- level of inflammation in the body decreases
- tissues have time to repair
- insulin and leptin sensitivity is improved
- important preventive measure against diabetes

Not Everything Is about Obesity—but a Lot Is

Remember that fasting has very little in common with pure weight-loss methods. It isn't just about body weight, more about cleansing/protecting the body from the many various assaults from overindulgence (like postprandial inflammation, broken-down gut flora, and obesity-related illnesses). Yet, weight gain and obesity are strong reasons for recommending some form of fasting or structured eating. Acute illnesses, not least cerebral hemorrhage or cardiac infarct, often happen in connection with large meals and important food holidays. Incidents of illness and mortality increase drastically at Christmas, New Year's, and Easter, and emergency rooms at hospitals are overrun. It puts a great burden on the body's organs when they receive those large amounts of sugar, sugar-like foods, and fat. Our bodies are, quite simply, not made to cope with this.

The following illnesses—all connected to the metabolism—have shown to have a strong association with obesity/elevated BMI. They can also be significantly counteracted by restricting calories (preferably permanently but also periodically).

- increased body inflammation
- too-elevated blood pressure
- excess blood fats—often called dyslipidemia (elevated "bad" cholesterol, LDL, low-density lipoprotein; too-low "good" cholesterol, HDL, high-density lipoprotein), too-numerous long-chain fatty acids
- type 2 diabetes
- acute and chronic heart disease
- brain hemorrhage
- gall and liver disease
- osteoarthritis
- sleep apnea and respiratory illnesses, including asthma
- certain cancers (especially uterus, breast, and colon cancer).

Nutrition Storage—the Fat Switch—and a Challenged Breakfast

Nutrition is stored three ways in the body: as sugar in liver and muscles, as abdominal fat, and as subcutaneous fat.

Obese individuals today carry a dangerously high amount of abdominal fat—about 13¼ pounds (6 kg)—and about 132¼ pounds (60 kg) in subcutaneous fat for someone weighing 265 pounds (120 kg). It is crucial to use up the fat instead of storing it.

Much information points to the conclusion that fat usage is not started until the sugar/glycogen is used up. For someone who wants to improve fat burning there is the 18/6 method. It is a version of time-restricted eating (TR) [also called intermittent fasting], where you let the metabolism rest for eighteen hours. Others prefer practicing general moderation in calorie consumption, that is, calorie restriction (CR).

Let's perform a mathematical example using the time-restricted method:

We assume that your last meal for the day is at 6 p.m. and that you have then replenished with 800 glycogen calories. With light physical occupation (reading or using the computer) you'll use up eighty-five calories per hour, which means that when you go to bed around 10:30 to 11:00 p.m., you have used up half of the calories. The calorie "burning" decreases to sixty-five calories per hour while you sleep, which means that your glycogen storage is completely empty by 5:00 a.m. Not until this hour does the fat "switch" turn from sugar mode to fat mode. However, from that hour, the fat switch needs another six hours without any calorie intake for the body to use and burn at least five hundred to six hundred calories.

It is common to rethink the necessity for breakfast if you follow these ideas (CR or TR), because breakfast, as a meal, has very little backing by research. To challenge breakfast among Westerners can start some very heated discussions.

Both CR and TR have shown to be successful in animal experiments, and more and more people practice the methods. Adolescents who sleep into late morning often have a time lapse in eating of fifteen hours or more.

This subject reminds me often of the Hunza people of Northern Pakistan. They go out into the fields at 5 a.m. on an empty stomach, return for their main meal at lunchtime, and then return to the fields again. As you already know, they manage on many fewer calories than what the health authorities in the West recommend. The Hunzas are seldom sick, and they are at the top of the list for the number of centenarians in the world.

To Structure Eating—a Lifestyle

It might be easier for some people to drop the evening meal instead of breakfast. Others prefer skipping breakfast. Either way there is room for a regularly performed half-day fast (intermittent fasting) according to the 18/6 principle. Simply speaking, the choice is between skipping breakfast and skipping dinner.

If you prefer to eat breakfast, choose something green and raw, for example, a green smoothie. The contents won't break down for about two to three hours, allowing organs to rest while fat burning continues. The fast is extended this way by two to three hours—the time it takes to transport the vegetables down to the gut bacteria, the only ones capable of breaking down such food. A glass of orange juice in the morning, however, will cancel the process immediately.

Calorie restriction (CR) is a variation with a stricter "eating principle." It is based on never eating to satiety. Instead, you eat and are satisfied with 2/3 of what you really would have liked. CR accomplishes the same health effects and good results as 18/6 intermittent fasting.

For many years, Marianne and I have practiced the CR method. We start the day with a beverage (mainly tea). We have our main meal at midday. It is a meal following the 80/10/10 method, similar to our ancestors' meal. We gladly add some deep-sea fish prepared on low heat. The evening meal is around 6 p.m. and is either a salad or a smoothie.

The old nutritional models like the food pyramid and the plate model are, in my opinion, long outdated. It is high time for new pedagogic models, perhaps in the style of 80/10/10? Just the way humans have eaten for millions of years and what our genes were developed with, before agriculture was introduced a few thousand years back. Do you feel that it sounds a bit meager? In that case, let me give you a tip—take a look at the dishes and recipes in this book. You can vary and season vegetables in many more ways than just always grating the same old carrots.

Our lifestyle choices determine if we want to stay healthy or be sick. This is true for most of us, to a high degree. We Westerners need to protect ourselves against overdoses of bad food.

> Practice daily intermittent fasting, that is, restrict your eating window to approximately six of the day's hours through practicing what is sometimes called skipping breakfast (no calories before lunch) or skipping dinner (no calories after 2 p.m.).
>
> FROM MY TWELVE COMMANDMENTS FOR OPTIMAL HEALTH, P. 74

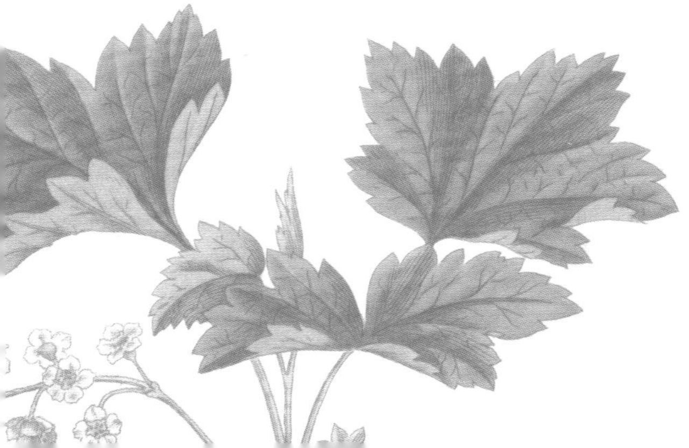

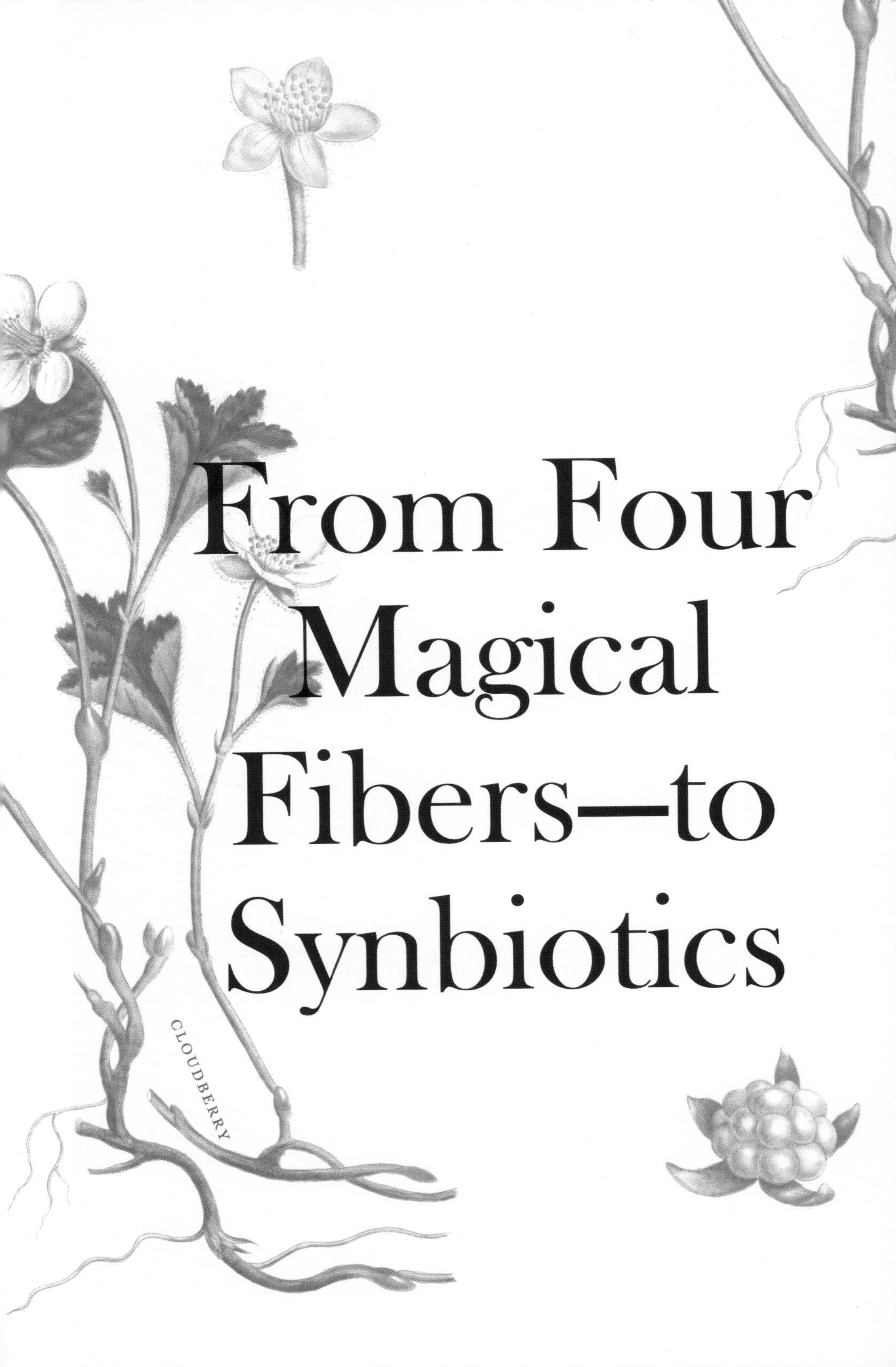

From Four Magical Fibers—to Synbiotics

10

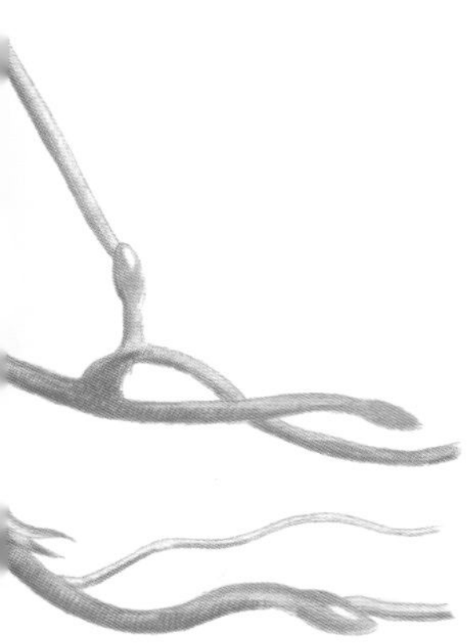

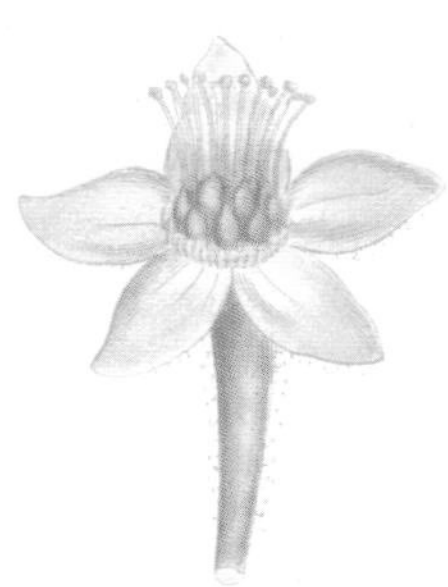

This chapter starts with a serious in-depth look at the importance of fibers in the intestinal tract. It also looks at the active role of bacteria in the metabolic process.

Then we go on to the true story of how, after many years of research, I succeeded in combining four magical fibers with a number of uniquely qualified lactobacilli.

The result is my particular composition within families of synbiotics—an effective remedy against IBS, kidney problems, and much more.

I haven't convinced everybody yet—but happily quite a few!

YOU ALREADY KNOW that fiber is food for our intestinal bacteria. You also know something about how the intestinal bacteria produce vital substances that strengthen our immune system and protect against illness.

While we wait for a rebirth of agriculture, food industry, and food habits, we have to search for all possible ways to enrich our food with plant fiber. Our ancestors ate 5¼ ounces (150 g) of pure plant fiber each day and had nearly double the rich intestinal flora we have today.

People in modern-day communities have lost their fiber-melting gut flora, matching how they have avoided "feeding" their bacteria.

When we live optimally and consume gut-friendly foods, we have around eight hundred to one thousand different kinds of good bacteria in our gut (altogether about 100 billion) that are fully occupied with extracting the thousands of wholesome elements we need for optimal health.

Apart from bacteria, there are other microorganisms in the gut, the roles of which are still largely unexplored. Most fibers can't be digested by our own enzymes in the stomach and small intestine, only by our "in-house" bacteria. which live primarily in the colon. So we have two digestive systems in succession, and both have to function properly. We can allow our colon to perform its important role if we carefully choose a bacteria-friendly diet, rich in various plant fibers and plant antioxidants.

The Gut—Our Afterburning Chamber

We have to go into more detail now.

Ideally an intestinal transit takes from twenty to twenty-four hours. A few hours after a meal, the plant fibers reach the colon, where they are digested in a "conveyor-belt system." The various bacteria have different and very specific tasks located in different regions within the colon. Some are situated at the very beginning of the colon and others at different distances from the anus. The bacteria working with the hardest-to-digest fibers, grains (mostly rye) for example, are located nearest the anus.

Even the most enthusiastic bacteria can't digest all fibers, and they leave them undigested. But these are nevertheless important, because they increase the volume of the stool and facilitate its passage out. The process to digest the fibers takes nearly twenty-four hours—a period when loads of energy and other beneficial substances are extracted and supplied to the body continually, carefully, and slowly. The colon has been likened to a plane's afterburning chamber—it "squeezes" as much energy as possible from the food.

Perhaps I don't reach 5¼ ounces (150 g) of plant fiber a day, but I pass the Blueberry test and the Kebnekaise [*] test with flying colors.

"The process to digest the fibers takes nearly twenty-four hours—a period when loads of energy and other nourishment is extracted continually, carefully, and slowly, then supplied to the body."

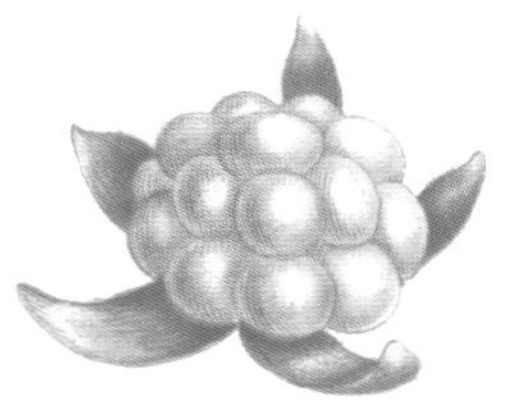

[*] Kebnekaise: Sweden's tallest mountain.

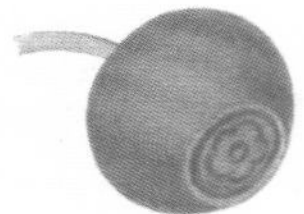

COLON FUNCTION—THREE SIMPLE TESTS YOU CAN TRY AT HOME

1

JERUSALEM ARTICHOKE TEST: The Jerusalem artichoke, just like garlic, onion, leeks, asparagus, artichokes, and bananas, is rich in good—but incredibly hard to digest—fibers called fructans. If you can eat a raw, average-sized Jerusalem artichoke in a salad, smoothie, or something similar without suffering digestive distress, you can be sure you have good intestinal flora.

2

KEBNEKAISE TEST: If your intestinal flora is working normally, it is common to pass large stools twice a day. Modern toilets are not built to accommodate Stone Age stools. If your stool reaches this size, a "mountaintop" will break the waterline.

3

BLUEBERRY TEST: Stone Age–imitating digestion needs about twenty hours between ingesting the meal and passing the stool. Lunch is passed between 8 and 9 a.m. the next morning, and the evening meal between midday and 1 p.m. You can check the correctness of this by keeping an eye out for when the blueberry appears.

THE MISSIONARY PHYSICIAN WHO DISCOVERED THE IMPORTANCE OF PLANT FIBERS

The British missionary physician Dennis Burkitt, who was stationed in Uganda in the twentieth century, was the first person who pointed to plant fibers' vital role in the intestine. He noted that the people living in the bush lacked most of the illnesses, both locally in the intestines (like appendicitis, inflammatory intestinal diseases, and cancer), but also in general, that the rest of humankind suffers from. His book *Don't Forget Fibre in Your Diet* was published in 1979 and became an international bestseller, opening the world's eyes to plant-fiber-rich foods.

Burkitt believed, in the beginning, that the explanation was in the large amount of raw and totally untreated plants that was part of the African diet, which hastened the passage through the intestine and contributed to toxins exiting the body faster. He, in due course, also realized the importance of introducing many benefits that bacteria could contribute.

He noted the amount of stool and the transit time from ingestion of food to defecation. He found the amount of stool in Europe was just over two ounces (60 g) per twenty-four hours—compared to the ten times larger amount in Uganda—approximately twenty-one ounces (600 g) per twenty-four hours. Transit time was about one hundred hours in Europe, compared with twenty hours in the African bush. At the same time other researchers observed that over half the patients in European long-term care had a transit time in excess of fourteen days!

Burkitt's observations brought humanity priceless knowledge. He received many rewards, but never a Nobel Prize. He was close, in fact, to getting a Nobel Prize in a different context when he discovered an earlier unknown form of tumor which is now named after him: "Burkitt's lymphoma."

THE BACTERIA CHEER, THE INTESTINE GRUMBLES

Many fibers can be consumed in large amounts; however, you have to be a bit more careful with others to give the intestines a chance to keep up.

Too much fiber can cause problems with gas, flatulence, bloating, and pain. It is called IBS (irritable bowel syndrome) when it becomes chronic—we will soon touch on this subject. Australian researchers have brought out a list, for IBS sufferers and many others, called FODMAP. It lists which fibers to be careful with and which fibers you can eat plenty of.

It's estimated that about half the population of North America, Australia, and Europe suffers from various digestive ailments. People suffering from these problems are therefore recommended to avoid "tough" fibers, or at least reduce their consumption of these. They are told to focus on eating the "kinder" fibers. I, personally, have different and more fun plans to propose: cooperate with your intestines, develop raw food eating, and add synbiotics if needed.

The FODMAP foods (which contain a lot of "tough" fiber and some which certain individuals are advised to refrain from eating) are these: apple, apricot, blackberries, dried fruit, figs, mango, nectarine, papaya, peaches, pears, plums, watermelon, cauliflower, artichoke, mushrooms, and peas.

Low-FODMAP foods (with lower amount of "tough" fibers, and which can be consumed freely) are, among others: bananas, blueberries, cantaloupe, cranberries, grapes, kiwi, lemon, lime, mandarins, oranges, passion fruit, pineapple, raspberries, rhubarb, strawberries, tangerines; as well as the vegetables alfalfa, bamboo shoots, Spanish pepper, carrots, cucumber, eggplant, green beans, kale, lettuce, parsnips, pumpkin, potatoes, radishes, seaweed, spinach, squash, tomatoes, turnip, zucchini, quinoa. However, most of these are rich in fructose, which is a reason for certain moderation.

I will return to my criticism of the FODMAP guidelines.

A Fiber Quartet with Magic Effects

There are thousands and thousands of fibers in the plant world. There are both beneficial and harmful fibers, but most of their health properties are still unexplored.

I have primary interest in four types of fibers that have absolutely magical health effects. I've been concentrating on these for more than fifteen years: pectin, inulin, beta-glucans, and resistant starch.

Let me introduce them to you!

PECTIN

Pectin is a true favorite, possibly also of the microbiome. One hundred percent of the pectin we eat will reach the colon and the bacteria.

Pectin is abundant in green unripe bananas (a third of the fruit's fiber is pectin); it is also found in apple (mostly concentrated in the peel), various citrus fruits (mostly in the peel); likewise in plums, grapes, cherries, cranberries, blueberries, gooseberries, quince, red and blackcurrants, apricots, blackberries, raspberries, strawberries, and peaches.

This fiber has a unique ability to reduce metabolic syndrome and significantly reduce the level of harmful (LDL) cholesterol in the blood.

Fruit pectin forms a jelly, which makes some of the fruits suitable for making jams and marmalades. Pectin also reduces the amount of additional sugar needed; if you freeze the jam and marmalade, you hardly need any additional sugar at all.

Pectin has also shown to have wide-ranging beneficial effects in several diseases. Its ability to stick to damp surfaces gives it the unique capability to protect mucous membranes and to carry medications to affected areas, all the way from nose to anus.

We showed in tests twenty-five years ago that green bananas were just as effective as that time's best drug, Astra's Losec. That time it was all about preventing/healing stomach ulcers and acid reflux. Unripe bananas are also excellent to quickly reduce diarrhea and vomiting and are used frequently in developing countries with individuals as young as infants of six months all the way into geriatric care.

In a smaller study, pectin showed to effectively inhibit the growth of prostate cancer when no other treatments were effective.

> "We showed in tests twenty-five years ago that green bananas were just as effective as that time's best drug, Astra's Losec."

To receive clinical effects from pectin, it needs to be consumed in large quantities daily—at least 1/5 ounce (6 g), the equivalent of approximately four grapefruits—or very large amounts of other pectin-rich fruits and berries.

Known health-promoting effects of pectin:

- lowers dramatically LDL cholesterol in the blood
- blood thinning
- counteracts diseases like diabetes, atherosclerosis, and cerebral hemorrhage. (Experimental studies suggest that the size of the hemorrhage is significantly smaller if pectin is given.)

INULIN

Inulin is, by far, the most studied fiber for its health effects. There are about 11,000 research papers on inulin to look into.

Inulin belongs to the carbohydrate group fructans. The highest level is found in chicory, Jerusalem artichoke (⅕ of the root is actually pure inulin), garlic (9 to 16% is inulin), leeks (3 to 10% is inulin), stewing onions (2 to 6% is inulin), red onions, and many other varieties of onions. Bananas also have inulin content, even if the level is very small (0.3% to 0.7%). You'll find inulin in asparagus and dandelion roots, too.

Here are a few examples of inulin's beneficial effects, chosen from an abundance of research papers:

The person who can cope with a certain amount of intestinal distress can count on that both total amount and variety of gut bacterial strains increase appreciably according to a study in which thirty overweight women were given a rather large daily dose of

½ oz (16 g) of inulin for three months. The increase in variety of bacterial strains was dramatic.

Inulin increases insulin sensitivity, decreases metabolic syndrome, and counteracts type 2 diabetes. Forty volunteers with type 2 prediabetes were given a large dose—1 ounce (30 g)—of inulin for two weeks and showed a dramatic decrease in blood glucose levels.

A large part of our population has unfortunately lost the gut bacteria that are able to digest these wholesome fibers. If they eat more than 1⁄10 ounce (2 to 3 g) of inulin a day, they will suffer from gastric distress like gas, bloating, and nausea. It is really regrettable because there probably doesn't exist another fiber that can confer so many health benefits.

An everyday use of onions, for example, is nothing to worry about. "A day without an onion is a lost day!" Eat it raw or lightly steamed.

The banana has, despite its slight content of inulin, shown itself to be able to inhibit and protect against development and return of various inflammatory gastric ailments.

BETA-GLUCANS

There's an abundance of beta-glucans in brewer's yeast, various mushrooms (such as shiitake, maitake, reishi, shimeji, and oyster mushrooms), and especially in oats. The latter explains why oat is so often lauded as exceptionally healthy. The amount eaten doesn't have to be restricted. I'm tempted to say the more the better. You'll find beta-glucans in barley and dates, too.

Beta-glucans demonstrate such an important and definite effect at decreasing bad cholesterol in the blood that the authorities in the United States allow it to be marketed with the phrase: "may reduce risk of heart disease." An intake of only 1⁄10 ounce (3 g) beta-glucans from oats has been shown to reduce the bad blood cholesterol by as much as 23 percent.

Apart from its heart-protecting effects, beta-glucans have shown in studies that they:

- protect against antibiotic-resistant strains of bacteria
- protect against cancer, such as, for example, melanoma
- increase energy, improve mood, and protect against infections—especially influenza and particularly in stressed women. (Studies show that supplementing with this fiber reduces the instance of infections by ⅔.)

RESISTANT STARCH

This fiber is called resistant starch because 100 percent of this fiber goes directly to the colon without being broken down by the body's own enzymes in the stomach or small intestine. The breakdown can only be performed by the microbiota in the colon. There are four kinds of resistant starch:

- RS1—the fiber is locked in the bran and can only be released by bacteria: grains, seeds, legumes.
- RS2—potatoes, sweet potatoes, unripe banana—an important fiber that turns into starch/sugar if cooked.
- RS3—RS1 and RS2 fibers which when they are allowed to cool will return to resistant starch (recrystallization). This capacity is maintained also when reheating carefully—not over normal body temperature.
- RS4—an industrially manufactured synthetic form, for example, high-maize resistant starch.

Resistant starch is one of fibers' unknown quantities. It is possibly the main source for production of an intestinal sealant, benefiting both weight and the intestinal system, and inflammation-lowering short-chain fatty acids (primarily butyric acid) known to counteract metabolic syndrome. Resistant starch is also known to counteract obesity.

Daily consumption of ½ to 1 ounce (15 to 30 g) has, according to a study, shown to effectively counteract metabolic syndrome while at the same time contribute at least 10 percent weight loss in obese individuals.

There's an abundance of resistant starch in green bananas, raw potatoes, and other root vegetables; as well as in peas, beans, lentils, grains, and seeds.

Resistant starch reaches the colon intact, where it is digested and releases nutrients and other wholesome substances. As a result:

- type 2 diabetes is counteracted through increased sensitivity and sparing of insulin
- levels of both blood glucose and insulin are decreased
- creation of butyric acid is increased. Butyric acid is important nourishment for the intestinal wall.
- the butyric acid seals the intestinal wall and stops leakage of toxins and bacteria into the body
- the immune system is strengthened
- the grade of inflammation is lowered

IBS—the Most Common Disease Globally?

Before I continue to talk about my work for a functioning combination of fibers and bacteria, I would like to describe the problem affecting a very large group, namely the already mentioned sufferers of IBS. It describes very clearly how the need for *ecobiologicals* (in my case, my synbiotics combination) might look:

Irritable bowel syndrome (IBS) is largely a disease of middle age. It's estimated that every fourth working adult in the West is a sufferer. Two thirds are women (and they are also worst affected) and a third men. About 40 percent of all sufferers have a milder version of IBS, while 35 percent have a reasonably tolerable version, but 25 percent suffer from a difficult and incredibly debilitating version of the illness.

The basic complaint with IBS is "a sore gut," a problem that more often than not gets worse after a meal, and then gets better a while after passing stool. The bathroom visits don't follow a pattern, but are highly irregular. The complaints come and go and are absent periodically. Bloating, flatulence, rumbling, and urgency are part of the symptoms. The stool's consistency varies daily between solid and loose: a hard lump may be followed by diarrhea-like stool. There's often a feeling of never really emptying the colon, so the sufferers visit the bathroom often and with frequent wiping.

The problem is physicians cannot diagnose IBS without first eliminating more serious diagnoses, like cancer, in any of the abdominal organs.

THIS WEIGHS HEAVILY ON THE COMMUNITY AND THE INDIVIDUAL

It ought to be possible to diagnose an IBS sufferer immediately, but that is not the case. It's reported it takes, on average, five physician visits before the diagnosis is made.

IBS sufferers use double the number of sick days compared with others taking sick leave. It is estimated to cost American society a minimum of $21 billion just in work absenteeism.

"It's reported that it takes, on average, five physician visits before the diagnosis is made."

Women are the hardest hit because they are often subjected to unnecessary surgical interventions like appendix removal, sometimes even a full hysterectomy, in the effort to get rid of their abdominal troubles. Often the patients have also been given unnecessary antibiotics, in the hope that this course would control the complaint at least temporarily. Strangely enough, it does seem to have helped occasionally.

IBS is often present together with other conditions such as lactose and gluten sensitivity. So, in the past, a lactose and/or gluten-free diet could help to provide some relief.

Lately, however, a connection has been identified between a deficiency in processing the especially hard-to-digest plant fibers fructans—an umbrella term for fibers of monosaccharide, oligosaccharide, or polysaccharide character. That's where FODMAP enters the picture with the list of hard-to-digest foods that I referred to earlier. Unfortunately, even a strict adherence to a FODMAP-reduced regimen doesn't help everybody. About 25 percent still experience continuing problems. The FODMAP list is far from complete. Long lists of other plants are also rich in fructans, among them the grains wheat, rye, and barley just as potatoes and all the ones listed here:

> Apple, pear, peach, mango, watermelon, canned and bottled fruit, dried fruit, honey, juice, wheat and rye in larger quantity (bread, pasta, biscuits), broccoli, Brussels sprouts, white cabbage, onion, garlic, peas, legumes, apple, apricot, cherries, nectarines, plums, avocado, mushrooms, cauliflower, artificial sweeteners (for example, sorbitol, xylitol and mannitol)

Many of these "forbidden" vegetables have been rated especially wholesome through the years, especially the ones richest in fructans, such as unripe banana, onion, garlic, and also Jerusalem artichoke.

So how will all Westerners suffering from digestive problems find the correct solution and get their gut microbiome regenerated?

The Solution Is Synbiotics

Only a handful of the gut's bacteria can digest fructans. A lot points to the fact that today's Westerners have never been "colonized" with these "specialists"; or they have early on lost them because they have deprived them of "work/food." Quite simply, they have not consumed a fructan-rich diet.

The solution was presented in 1994 by Marina Müller and Dorothee Lier, researchers from an agriculture research facility in Braunsweig, Germany. They were researching animal feed preservation (ensilage). Incomplete breakdown/decomposition of fructans presented a problem for long-term storage of animal feed. Müller and Lier tested no fewer than 712 strains of lactobacilli, all of them recuperated from plant matter, mostly grass.

"Only a handful of the gut's bacteria can digest fructans."

Read and be bowled over: Only sixteen of these lactobacillus strains could break down phlein, a fructan with no fewer than five bindings. Only eight could digest inulin, which is perhaps the best-known and currently most used prebiotic.

These lactobacillus are identified through their full names as *Lactobacillus paracasei* subsp. *sparacasei*, *Lactobacillus plantarum*, *Lactobacillus brevis*, and *Pediococcus pentosaceus*. Three of these are included in my new synbiotic mixture (though not the same strains). All the strains of *Lact. paracasei* subsp. *paracasei* tested showed the ability to digest fructans. It was a bit more difficult for other lactobacilli. Most of the tried strains except two of *L. plantarum* had more difficulty in digesting inulin than phlein.

As we know, the basic problem is our gut microbiome has slowly thinned, and this impoverishment continues today. We knew this nearly forty years ago without doing anything about it worth mentioning. The problem was made clear in 1983 by the eminent American microbiologist Steven Finegold. This could later be confirmed by my team of colleagues around what would become Probi, which we started on at the end of 1990.

Early on it was clear, just the fructan that was fermenting lactobacillus *L. plantarum* and *L. paracasei* had suffered the most from the microbiome's impoverishment. In other words, it was not by chance that it was a *L. plantarum* strain that became Probi's star bacteria. It continues to be even today, and the health beverage Proviva is built around it.

A NEW IDEA: FIBERS ARE "TRAVEL FOOD" FOR THE BACILLUS

Personally, I wanted to continue with the research, but the structure of the Probi company didn't allow for this at the time. I wanted, primarily, to focus on searching for new lactobacilli—not the ones from the human impoverished intestine but in nature, just like Müller and Lier had done.

Another ambition pushed me to add nourishing fibers (prebiotics) to the chosen lactobacillus— "travel food" for the trip down to their final workstation, the colon. We choose to add the four "magical" fibers I told you about, of which one, inulin, was a fructan. The combination pre- and probiotics, presently called synbiotics, are well known today for their powerful health-promoting effects.

Through this new approach, my colleagues and I eventually found several lactobacillus with unexpectedly strong immune functions. Three of them became part of the new synbiotics that I've arrived at in my research: *Plantarum, Paracasei*, and *Pediococcus*. The final product of my research was given the brand name Synbiotic 2000.

The bacteria that Marina Müller and Dorthee Lier discovered having unique digestive capabilities are now well-established as probiotics, and they are part of my own blend. These two female scientists were extremely inspirational for my work. They deserve a Nobel Prize if it turns out that they also found the key to one of the world's most troublesome "scourges"—IBS.

I continue to look for answers to questions that pop up at the front of my own research: Obese people are nearly totally lacking in fructan-fermenting *L. Paracasei* and *Plantarum*. Are fructan foods less obesity-promoting? Obesity often goes hand in hand with IBS; what connections are still undiscovered?

THROW THE FODMAP LIST IN THE WASTEPAPER BASKET!

Medical wisdom today says it is certainly sensible to avoid certain plant matter—"FODMAP to feel good." But there is still nothing there which looks like a basic approach of eating enough plants to produce a healthy gut microbiome.

My advice is: Throw the FODMAP list in the wastepaper basket!

Additionally, I tell curious researchers/physicians and current patients alike: Search high and low for the fructan-digesting bacteria a big portion of humankind has lost. They exist everywhere around you in the plant world. They are there to protect and nourish the plant that harbors them. They can change the lives of severely afflicted IBS sufferers, worn-out dialysis-dependent individuals, and many more.

While waiting to discover these bacteria, feel free to use the ones in my synbiotics product. How much to take is individual, you'll have to test your way. Be patient, it might take several months before you see any result.

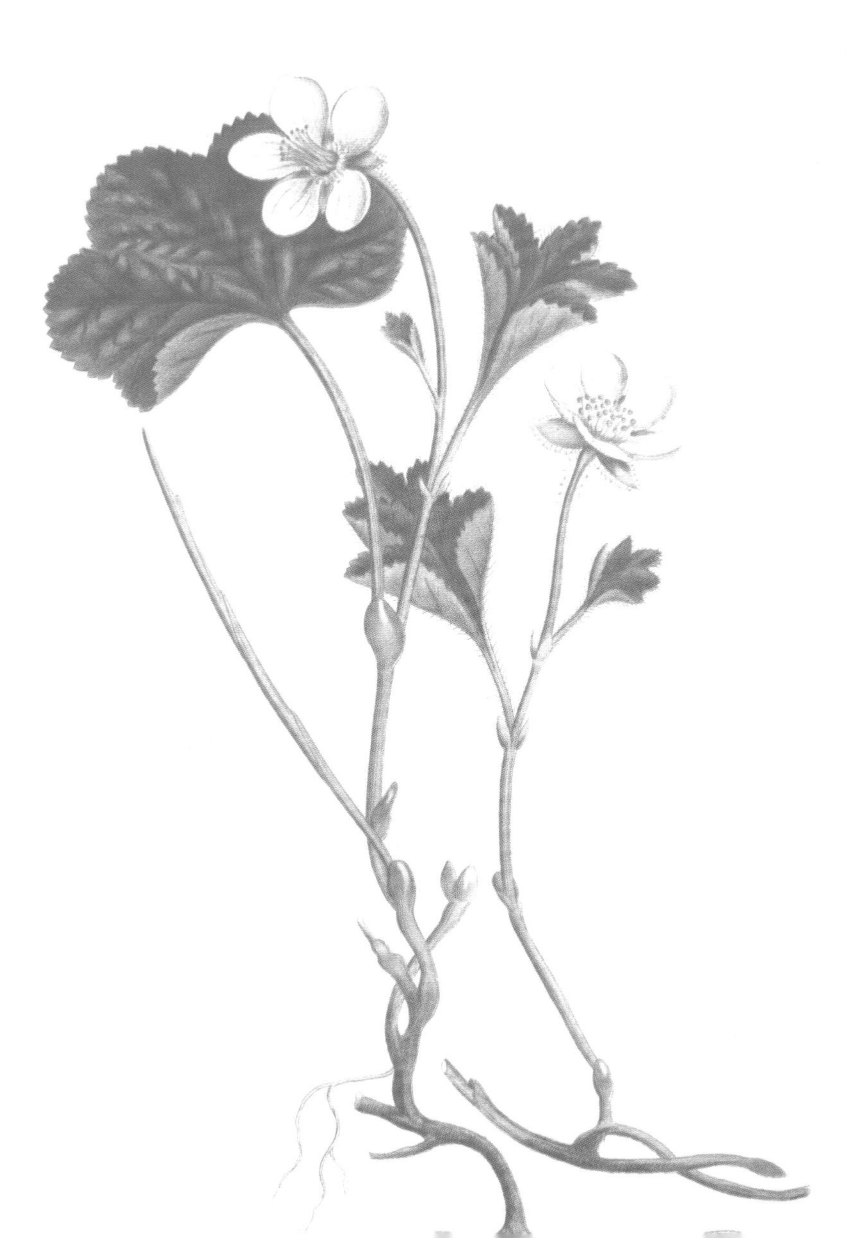

With Warm Greetings to Swedish Healthcare

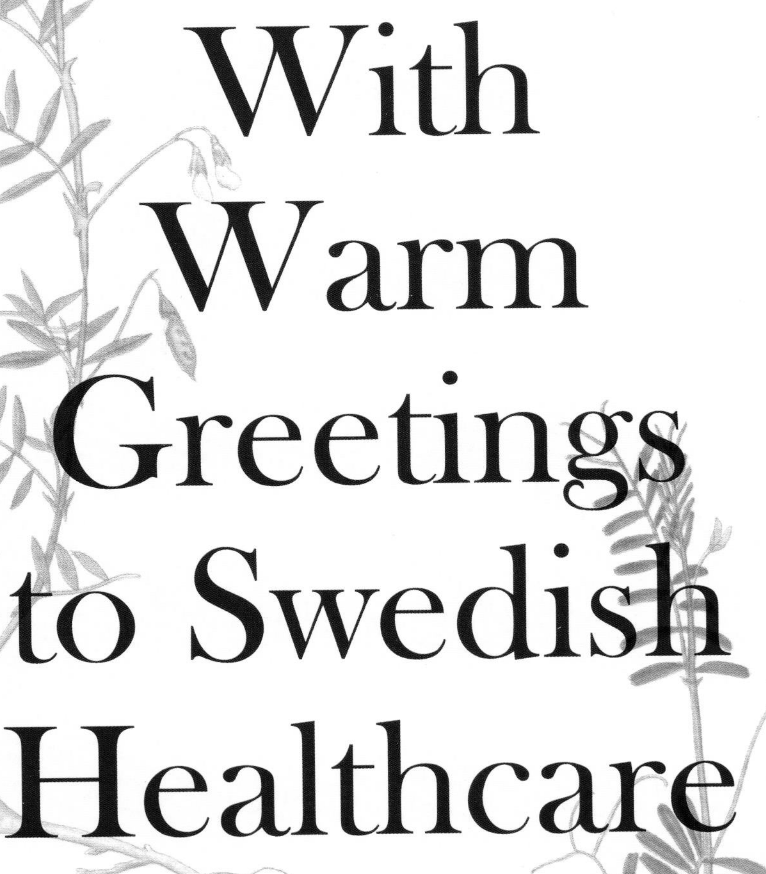

PEA PLANT

11

Healthcare thinking needs reinvention in many ways, not just to deal with the enormous overburden that threatens to collapse it from within. The need is pressing because many of our common illnesses demand completely different treatments than the traditional "diagnosis-and-pharmaceutical"-based methods.

Bring in the eco-biologic outlook to the patients who are only offered inferior alternatives. Reintroduce preventive care—attack health problems before people head into chronic illness. Work in symbiosis with wellness coaches and other new professions, and accept co-responsibility for a more healthy lifestyle.

Last but not least: acknowledge the individuals' increased responsibility for their own health and especially intestinal health!

HISTORICALLY, MEDICAL CARE was developed with the hope it would make a lot of surgery redundant. These dreams have only marginally been realized.

Another dream, and this one seems to have totally disintegrated, is the one about government healthcare being responsible for preventive care. I participated in one of the governmental advisory committees that initiated the community health centers in Sweden. One of the main tasks of the health centers was to inform and educate about health and actively work at preventive healthcare. Hundreds of community health centers were established. However, no preventive efforts were initiated. The situation remains the same today. No community health center will pay for, let's say, a test for vitamin D deficiency unless there is already a visible sign of deficiency.

What is worse, the community health centers are mainly occupied with picking up overload from other health services and have few possibilities to put into practice their own preventive health care. A government minister told me a few years ago: "That is not part of community responsibility." Is it up to each individual? In this way, society has to pay for people's unhealthy living. In the end it is probably more expensive than preventive healthcare.

The Pharmaceutical Industry Is a Huge Brake Shoe

Today's medical care is recognized (and weighed down?) primarily by its association with a new industry heavyweight, the enormous and moneyed pharmaceutical industry. Coming in with my "alternative medicine" label, as developer of symbiotic supplements, I have had to continuously bow and scrape to be allowed to do clinical studies in the healthcare setting. Sometimes the jargon has been openly hostile and pretty cynical.

"Are you really that stupid? To think that I would test your pills, so they can end up putting our own drugs out of business?"

There certainly is a true and honest belief in chemical drugs, and it's probably justified to a certain degree. However, there is a solid rallying around the pharmaceutical companies that prevents an unbiased discussion—especially around chemical drugs' harmful effects on the gut microbiome.

An old colleague of mine said recently, apropos something I had written about the risks of certain drugs:

"Imagine, Stig, that we have to reach retirement age before we dare speak up about the situation."

Fortunately, there have always existed independent thinkers within healthcare who have met my colleagues and me with openness and interest. Nurses have always been the first to stick their neck out! For example, I remember how they gladly introduced the new health beverage Proviva on the wards, because they quite simply deemed the beverage did the patients a lot of good.

BRILLIANT SUCCESS FOR SYNBIOTICS— THE EU WANTS TO FORBID THE CONCEPT

As time passes, a diversity of representatives from the healthcare system have shown increasing interest and respect for my research.

For example, at the legendary Charité hospital in Berlin, Germany, a larger study was made of my synbiotics on their own initiative. They showed great success in 2004 for the synbiotics among liver-transplant patients. It was so great the outside world had difficulty taking it all in.

Infections after transplants were practically eliminated, and identifiable bacteria outside the intestines decreased by 97.5 percent. Antibiotic use decreased 97 percent. Patient stay in the ICU reduced to 1.4 days from 8.8 days!

You would think that my synbiotic product would be used everywhere fourteen years later. Alas, that's not the case at all. The bureaucracy is enormous, and many permits are needed.

"They showed great success in 2004 for the synbiotics among liver-transplant patients."

MY COMMENT: The pharmaceutical industry's stubborn opposition to ecobiologic supplements has strong support in Europe. Just as this is being written, the EU is preparing, not surprisingly, to try to forbid the designations probiotics and synbiotics. What doesn't healthcare stand to lose by being so dependent on chemical drugs which wreak so much havoc in the intestine? What won't the patients lose by having to forgo precious, proven alternatives to the chemical, often toxic, substances?

Minimize Contact with Chemicals. Avoid All Nonessential Pharmaceuticals and Only Use Drugs for Internal or External Use When They Are Absolutely Necessary.

FROM MY TWELVE COMMANDMENTS FOR OPTIMAL HEALTH, P. 74

Chronic Kidney Sufferers Are Left Out in the Cold

I'll give an in-depth example of the unnecessary opposing stances between classical medicine and alternative medicine. I wish to show how difficult it can be to get clinical trials going with natural supplements, even though there are plenty of studies pointing to the patients as the winners.

This case is from Swedish kidney care.

Here is the scientific starting point: In order to have good health, it is vital the gut bacteria effectively contribute to breaking down consumed proteins. This produces a release of uremic toxins (in the urine) which otherwise would create a large burden for our kidneys. The chronic kidney disease patient lacks this protective mechanism and therefore belongs to an especially vulnerable group. In addition, it's in this matter precisely that their dialysis treatment is not sufficient.

We normally expect the microbiota will thoroughly reduce the inflammation in the body, increase the efficiency of our own immune system, and indirectly protect against repeat infections, chronic illnesses, and premature aging.

Patients suffering from chronic kidney disease (often shortened ESRD—end-stage renal disease; also terminal kidney failure) always lack a well-functioning microbiota. This also applies to sufferers of other illnesses, such as Alzheimer's disease, ADHD, diabetes, COPD (chronic obstructive pulmonary disease), and chronic liver disease.

It's my opinion all these individuals should always receive supplemental synbiotics.

THE LIMITS OF DIALYSIS

Dialysis is admittedly a very effective way to remove many of the toxins that daily build up in the body, especially PD (peritoneal dialysis). This newer method allows continuous cleaning done through only a change of abdominal fluid.

However, as already mentioned, all dialysis methods have their limits, and the procedure is far from as effective as we could wish. It is well known that the dialysis patient suffers from high levels of oxidative stress, clearing the road for cardiovascular disease, metabolic syndrome, weight loss/anorexia, anemia, and other complications. Even chronic fatigue is especially common in this group.

Often found in the blood of hemodialysis patients are not only uremic toxins, but also whole or part of intestinal bacteria, as well as many malignant bacteria. A study showed DNA from harmful intestinal bacteria in at least 20 percent of the group's hemodialysis patients.

The primary goal of dialysis is to identify and eliminate "organic garbage products." Approximately ninety to one hundred such "garbage products" have been identified. However, reports show that the leakage of bacterial toxins is much larger in patients receiving hemodialysis than the ones going through peritoneal dialysis.

The intestinal problems of the chronic kidney disease patient have been known for decades.

Against this background, it's inconceivable not many efforts have been made to try to recondition the intestines, decrease the production of toxins, and stop the leakage of bacterial toxins in the body.

"The intestinal problems of the chronic kidney disease patient have been known for decades."

LIMITED STUDIES—POSITIVE RESULTS

A small study, which gave promising results, was performed already in probiotics' infancy. Eight hemodialysis patients were given *Lactobacillus acidophilus*, lactic acid bacteria, which are common in yogurt. The treatment effectively reduced the toxin dimethylamine (DMA) in the blood. A 50 percent reduction in the blood of the carcinogen toxin nitrosodimethylamine was also seen.

Later studies show that a daily supplementation with a very small dose, ⅓ to ⅔ ounce (10–20 g), of prebiotic fibers significantly reduces the amount of the bacterial toxin p-Cresol sulfate in the blood. This can be compared with the synbiotic composition I arrived at, which contains ⅓ ounce (10 g) of specific prebiotic fibers.

It would take fifteen years before the publication of another study. This time a synbiotic concoction was tried. Even though there were evident limits in the study's execution, it still showed significantly lower levels of the toxin p-Cresol sulfate in the blood, and a decreased level of constipation. Unfortunately, no flood of studies of more specific pro- and synbiotic preparations followed this time either.

META-ANALYSIS SHOWS UNIQUE POSSIBILITIES

The first meta-analysis—an analysis of everything published to that date—about supplementation of pre-, pro-, and synbiotics to dialysis patients was published in 2012.

Despite the aforementioned studies' restrictions, they show strong indications that synbiotic treatment effectively reduces the blood levels of the bacterial toxins indoxyl sulfate and p-Cresol sulfate.

A study from 2015 provides great hope. During a six-month period, thirty-nine patients were given either a probiotic or a placebo. The kidney function was better preserved in the probiotic-treated group.

I work personally with much larger doses.

New filters have facilitated more effective dialysis treatment, but there remain considerable problems. The inability of dialysis to eliminate these toxins is far from what one wishes.

SYNBIOTICS' POTENTIAL IN END-STAGE DISEASE

Treatment with synbiotics is a great option for eliminating a very distressing fatigue often observed in dialysis patients and sometimes also in transplant patients.

According to the researcher Tammy L. Sirich and colleagues, there exist a number of nearly unidentifiable protein-bound toxins that dialysis is not very effective at eliminating; their clinical effects are far from clarified.

Synbiotic treatment is focused on the elimination of just such protein-bound toxins and can therefore become an important adjunct to an otherwise successful dialysis treatment during end-stage kidney disease.

I have tried for at least fifteen years, to no avail, to pursue clinical studies with synbiotics for kidney patients. I have visited, lectured, and tried to interest nephrologists the world over, from leading clinics in Stockholm and London to so-called developing countries.

The enthusiasm has not been lacking among the nephrologists. However, at the last minute a large pharmaceutical company or similar institution paying large sums comes up with an "absolutely vital" tryout for a new drug, new filter, or some such thing.

MY COMMENT: I'm absolutely convinced that kidney care—probably just as overburdened as most care units—would have an easier workload if their patients did get an opportunity to use synbiotics and improve their intestinal workings in a totally harmless way.

A Drastic Increase in ADHD Is Trying the Healthcare System

As mentioned earlier, the WHO has reported the number of chronic illnesses has increased very rapidly in the last half century, especially noninfectious illness. This applies even to youth in the age-group of three to seventeen years; it is estimated that 15 percent in this age group already suffer from some kind of chronic disease.

This increase is assumed to be in great part because of all the chemicals added to our foods (more than three hundred at the moment). It is disconcerting to read that the occurrence of autism in the United States has increased by 290 percent in just over ten years (1997–2008), and ADHD by 33 percent. The global trend is similar, including Sweden.

In Sweden, the number of children diagnosed with ADHD is reported to have risen approximately 700 percent over the last ten years. The example is taken from Västmanland's county, but the same trend can be seen in the whole country. It is possible that the increase is even larger—there is a lot of underreporting.

CONVENIENCE FOODS ARE SUSPECTED

ADHD is associated with low birth weight (below 5½ pounds [2½ kg]). According to a British study looking at approximately 20,000 subjects, although with many exceptions, ADHD is strongly overrepresented in groups with so-called socioeconomic problems: low income, poverty, young mothers, parents' lack of education, single parenthood, etc. ADHD in the young age-group is described as the gateway to socioeconomic problems and big health concerns also later in life, especially frequent drug abuse. Lack of knowledge about food and health was also observed in this group.

Even though ADHD's basic cause is in many ways still very much unclear, more and more of today's researchers associate the disease with lifestyle-related factors, and especially to the chemical additives in convenience foods.

We recently mentioned how substandard information about food additives is on packaging. Hurried individuals, especially parents with small children (who might need to use convenience foods), probably have extra difficulties following these "warnings." To stop buying convenience foods seems to be the best alternative for ADHD families. This is what the majority of researchers recommend.

MY COMMENT: The ADHD problem shows extremely vividly that the healthcare system must resume responsibility for preventive care.

> "Minimize contact with bacterial toxins, such as endotoxins, as well as different environmental toxins."
>
> FROM MY TWELVE COMMANDMENTS FOR OPTIMAL HEALTH, P. 74

A Hunt in the Dark for Toxins

The ADHD challenge leads us directly into the unchecked turmoil that the flourishing toxins constitute for each individual.

It is a very unsafe feeling to know that we are all exposed to many hundreds, probably thousands, of chemical substances and that the health consequences of these are far from being examined closely. Some of them aren't even completely known.

The EU stated in a report twenty years ago that we have very little knowledge on about 90 percent of the chemicals humans are being exposed to. This was valid even if we only concerned ourselves with the chemicals that are used in larger quantities (more than 2,204,623 pounds per year).

The situation is hardly any better today—in fact, it's more like the opposite. A WHO report asserts the negative chemical impact on our health is actually a lot worse than we can imagine in our worst nightmare.

Pesticides are the environmental toxins that we have really paid the most attention to. There are several hundred approved pesticides in the EU and we, like the EU pointed out, don't know enough about their effect on our health. What's their half-life in the ground, in the water, and in the human body?

We are exposed to these substances several times each day and mainly in association with our meals. It is impossible to be completely protected against them, and the information about them is far too poor. Admittedly, there are laws both in the EU and Sweden stating that chemical additives must be declared on packaging. Unfortunately, these laws aren't followed as well as we would have expected. The information about additives is placed in an obscure place, in small print, and often in incomprehensible code.

The EU should have introduced mandatory reporting on pesticide content in fruit and vegetables, seeds, peas and beans, and wine a long time ago.

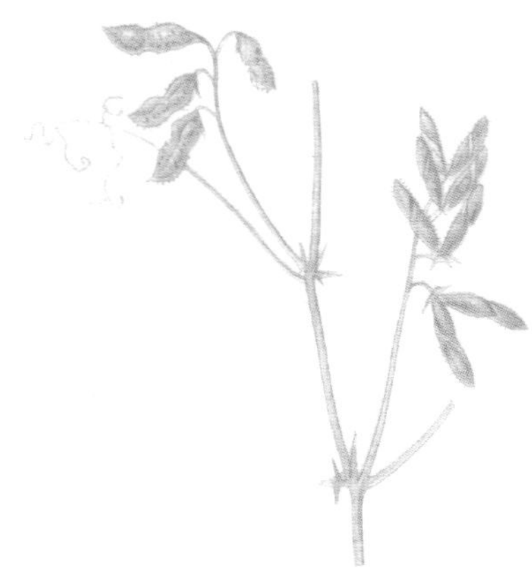

> "Reduce consumption of salt, both sodium and chloride. Increase intake of iodine. Use iodized salt, and avoid flour and bromine especially. Minimize contact with plastics and never heat plastic or plastic-covered items."
>
> FROM MY TWELVE COMMANDMENTS FOR OPTIMAL HEALTH, P. 74

OVERCONFIDENCE IN SAFE LIMITS

We are slowly starting to realize that it isn't just pesticides we have to keep an eye on. There is a long list of other products and substances shown to be much more harmful for our health than we really wanted to believe. Take, for example, silicone implants and colors in tattoos—substances that are placed on/in the skin or inside the body. These substances are known to travel in the body and affect our immune system. In medical literature, it is suspected that silicone from implants may contribute to the emergence of the "mysterious" illness fibromyalgia, as well as autoimmune diseases such as scleroderma.

It's not until recently that scientists have started to show greater interest in the so-called parabens and phthalates that are found in skin creams, soaps, makeup, scented candles, laundry detergents, toothpastes, and plastic toys. These substances, apart from affecting the immune system, have been shown to have troubling effects, especially on the thyroid gland, ovaries, and testicles. They are considered contributors for increased illness in these organs, with focus on reduced sperm count and increased infertility risk.

One of today's problems in our hunt for toxins is that too many people have overconfidence in the so-called safe limits. To stay below current safe limits for a certain substance induces a false sense of security. Different toxins have actually shown to enhance each other's effects. The result is a great inflammatory load on the body.

IT'S MURKY AROUND ORGANIC FOODS

Some convince themselves that organic food isn't just grown without artificial manure but also without pesticides. Is that true? Allow me to doubt.

When you dig deeper into the literature you'll find that organic pesticides (among them a rotenone pyrethrin mixture) are used in organic agriculture.

Researchers at Berkeley University in California compared organic grapes (sprayed on average seven to eight times per harvest with the rotenone pyrethrin mixture) with grapes used in traditional wine production (on average sprayed only twice per harvest with the synthetic product Imidan). They discovered the organic mixture with rotenone and pyrethrin was very likely more harmful for the environment (and health) than Imidan, especially if we take into account that the mixture has well-known negative effects primarily on fish, but also on other kinds of aquatic life in lakes and sea.

MY COMMENT: As for toxins, the responsibilities for more knowledge rests heavily on research itself. A specific responsibility of the healthcare system is to prevent harmful effects from synthetic drugs on the body. It is evident that the food industry has to speed up its pace of self-sanitizing against toxins. The public's increased interest in hunting down toxins is a force to be reckoned with.

Allergies Are Strongly Associated with Intestinal Health

Many call allergies an endemic Western disease, and it's often surrounded by a dejected impression that the reasons (and the remedies) are very difficult to find. This attitude is wholly out of date. We know much more today, and there are new ways to start out on prevention and cure.

An allergy is a well-known defense reaction when substances that usually don't belong in the body threaten one or several of the body's tissues/cells. Basically, it is an inflammation that expresses itself through redness, swelling, radiating heat, and lowered tissue function. The reaction is often visible on the skin, in the lungs, and the digestive system.

The digestive system is particularly exposed because any of the billions of different substances (allergens) that are introduced can cause an allergic reaction, and microorganisms might also create inflammation and infection. The combination of allergens and illness-generating bacteria is highly effective and undesirable.

> "If an individual doesn't get the chance to develop a gut flora and immune system the person will easily fall prey to allergies."

We know through animal tests that normal defense mechanisms can be thrown totally out of order if antibiotics or other kinds of chemicals are involved. This is exactly what is discovered in people who have mistreated their microbiome or have had it greatly reduced for other reasons.

A properly functioning gut microbiome is therefore a prerequisite for a strong defense against many different allergies.

A DIET OF PLANT MATTER IS THE ENEMY OF ALLERGIES

The incidence of serious and often life-threatening allergic reactions (anaphylactic shock) is unfortunately on the increase at an alarming rate. Even more "garden-variety" allergies are increasing rapidly, and today about 8 percent of children and 2 percent of all adults in the Western world suffer from some kind of allergy.

We get next to none of the "tough" fibers that are our gut flora's favorite foods. Least of all our children!

Admittedly, we have become attentive to the important allergy- and illness-inhibiting effects of certain substances that the gut flora produces locally on the surface of the intestinal mucosa, and especially in the first half of the colon.

The main problem here is that the "tough" fibers needed for this process have become too hard for many of us to digest. There just aren't any bacteria present any longer that are able to digest these fibers.

A reconditioning of the digestive system, in the form of suitable supplements, can be of help here.

PROBIOTICS CAN PREVENT

So far tests of probiotics against allergies have been mostly performed on animal subjects. Among observed results were strong inhibitory effects on the development of asthma in mice when given supplementation of lactobacillus.

Attempts have been made, if very cautiously, to try probiotics on human subjects. The results so far have been very varied; some bacteria have shown to be effective, others not. The administered doses varied too much and the size of the test groups that were treated was often too small. So far, no extra fiber was ever added simultaneously. The way things look currently, there is really no basis to recommend probiotics for different allergy manifestations; at least not to alleviate or cure allergies. However, this is a way to prevent the emergence of an allergy.

Without a doubt, it is obvious that a rich supply of short-chain fatty acids is necessary for optimal digestive health. We also know that allergic children have lower levels of propionic acid, acetic acid, and butyric acid in their gut compared with nonallergic children.

Obviously, the task is to try increasing the level of these important short-chain fatty acids in the gut using all means available. A bacterial composition rich in health-bringing fibers can hopefully contribute to this.

A POSITIVE SYNBIOTICS STUDY

Children with allergic skin changes (atopic dermatitis) run a great risk for also developing asthma. During a twelve-week study such children (average age was 17 months) were given a synbiotic combination of a small-dose bifidobacillus and a small dose of a mixture of galacto- and fructooligosaccharides—¼ ounce/3⅓ ounces (0.8 gr/100 ml)—as a prophylactic.

The treated children developed considerably fewer allergies.

After one year, 14 percent in the treated group showed signs of asthma compared with 34 percent in the control group, and 6 percent in the treated group had started on asthma medication compared with 26 percent in the control group. Five children in the control group had developed an observable allergy toward cats, something not seen in the synbiotic-treated group.

This small but partly inadequate investigation gives us hope that treatment with synbiotics can be substantially more effective than treatment with just probiotics. The treatment with synbiotics shouldn't be limited to just a few weeks, but rather given on a permanent basis; and the treatment should contain a larger amount of bacteria and fiber.

MY COMMENT: All our allergy sufferers deserve to try synbiotics. The long-term preventive work against allergies is just as vital—not least through a plant-based diet. Entice health coaches and nutritionists to join in this! My advice to expectant mothers, if followed, can have an effect on the health of many future children as a preventive measure to avoid allergies.

Can Synbiotics Replace Fecal Transplants?

In a well-functioning gut there ought to be 3⅓ to 4½ pounds (1.5–2 kg) of gut bacteria that make up a kind of "fecal organ," at least as big as the liver, which has loads of vital functions for our health. There ought to be at least ten times the amount of bacterial cells compared to our usual body cells, and each bacterium has its own specific function within the gut's conveyor-belt system.

It is not news for those who have read Guilia Ender's international bestseller *Gut: The Inside Story of Our Body's Most Underrated Organ*, that stool and evacuation habits are incredibly important for our health. Those who have read this far in *The Anti-Inflammatory Diet Solution* also recognize the major enemy of the fecal organ: processed Western foods. Raw foods fundamentalists and vegans can show brilliant results.

"High priority must therefore be given to the nurturing of your fecal organ with bacteria, and also to reconditioning if necessary."

Stress and added synthetic substances are also harmful for the fecal organ. All pharmaceutical drugs—antibiotics, hypertension medication, tranquilizers, stomach drugs, and sleeping pills—are in principle enemies of the "fecal organ." Chemotherapy drugs, commonly used in cancer treatment, are infamous for poisoning and strongly reducing the gut flora.

High priority must therefore be given to nurturing of your fecal organ with bacteria, and also to reconditioning if necessary.

Animals often eat feces, their own and that of other animals. Veterinarians have for centuries, and for various reasons, practiced the transfer of feces between different species. Treatment using feces has also been an important part of human medicine—for example, in Greek medicine about 2,500 years ago, long before anybody knew of the existence of bacteria.

With the growing problem of resistant strains of bacteria, fecal treatment is on the upswing again.

FECAL TRANSPLANTING IS ESTABLISHED

A good friend of mine, the surgeon Ben Eiseman (1917–2012), deserves to be honored for a pioneering effort. He treated patients with several enemas with donated stool. All of his six seriously ill patients recovered miraculously.

Of course, understandably, fecal transplants don't have a rustic appeal for either individuals or the permit-giving institutions. It took several decades before it was used again.

Today, however, it is evident that fecal transplants are a superior treatment form, especially when facing difficult conditions such as community-acquired *Clostridium difficile* infection (CDI), caused by one of the worst offenders among the bacterial strains. Here repeated treatments of what is called fecal microbiota transplantation (FMT) have shown to be very successful. Good donors are difficult to find, and no Westerner has an optimal fecal organ. However, repeated studies show that FMT is more effective than the alternative treatment with the antibiotic vancomycin, which often leads to recidivism as well, as causing irreparable damage to the "fecal organ" and the immune system. The authorities are understandably reluctant to relax the rules around FMT but have been forced to accept that FMT is used after two unsuccessful treatments with vancomycin.

Logically, donors ought to be recruited from individuals with especially rich fecal organs. Perhaps frozen stool from the South American Yanomami, from Hadzas, and from Burkina Faso will one day become a saleable commodity? In these cultures, people live like our ancestors did, and have more strains of bacteria than we have.

STRONG REASONS FOR SYNTHETIC FECAL MATTER

FMT has shown great success with exceedingly difficult chronic illnesses. Nevertheless, there are many undesirable components in donated stool. For that reason, before a transplant can take place, authorities demand a wide range of tests of both donor and recipient's fecal matter be performed. Even if very rare, it is possible to be infected by someone else's feces. According to everyone involved, FMT is also a "disgusting" treatment method. The motivation to find alternative and equivalent treatments is strong.

A laboratory-produced combination of effective bacteria and plenty of active fibers is therefore a very attractive alternative. That is exactly what my development of synbiotics is aiming for.

A step in the right direction: Ten patients with serious inflammation in the lower colon (distal colitis) were treated with synbiotics enemas. They were followed for three weeks, during which time all manifestations of the illness disappeared—frequency passing stool, amount of episodes of diarrhea, nightly diarrhea, blood in the stool. Even the consistency of the stool was thoroughly improved.

My hope is that my synbiotic composition will give as good results as FTM and, therefore, become a convenient and hygienic replacement for the time-consuming and not always very welcome fecal treatment method.

MY COMMENT: The progress of fecal transplants and, in the long term, synthetic stool (laboratory-fabricated fecal matter) shows how important cooperative experimentation is across scientific and administrative borders. Another example of how our ancestors were much more into health than we are!

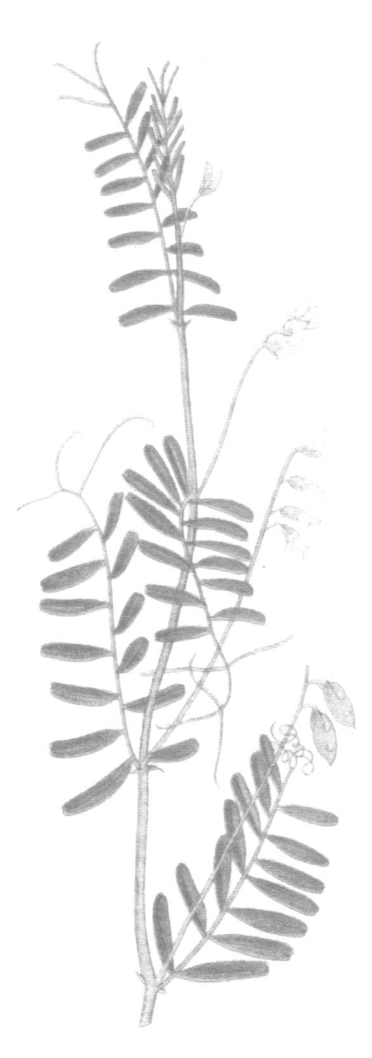

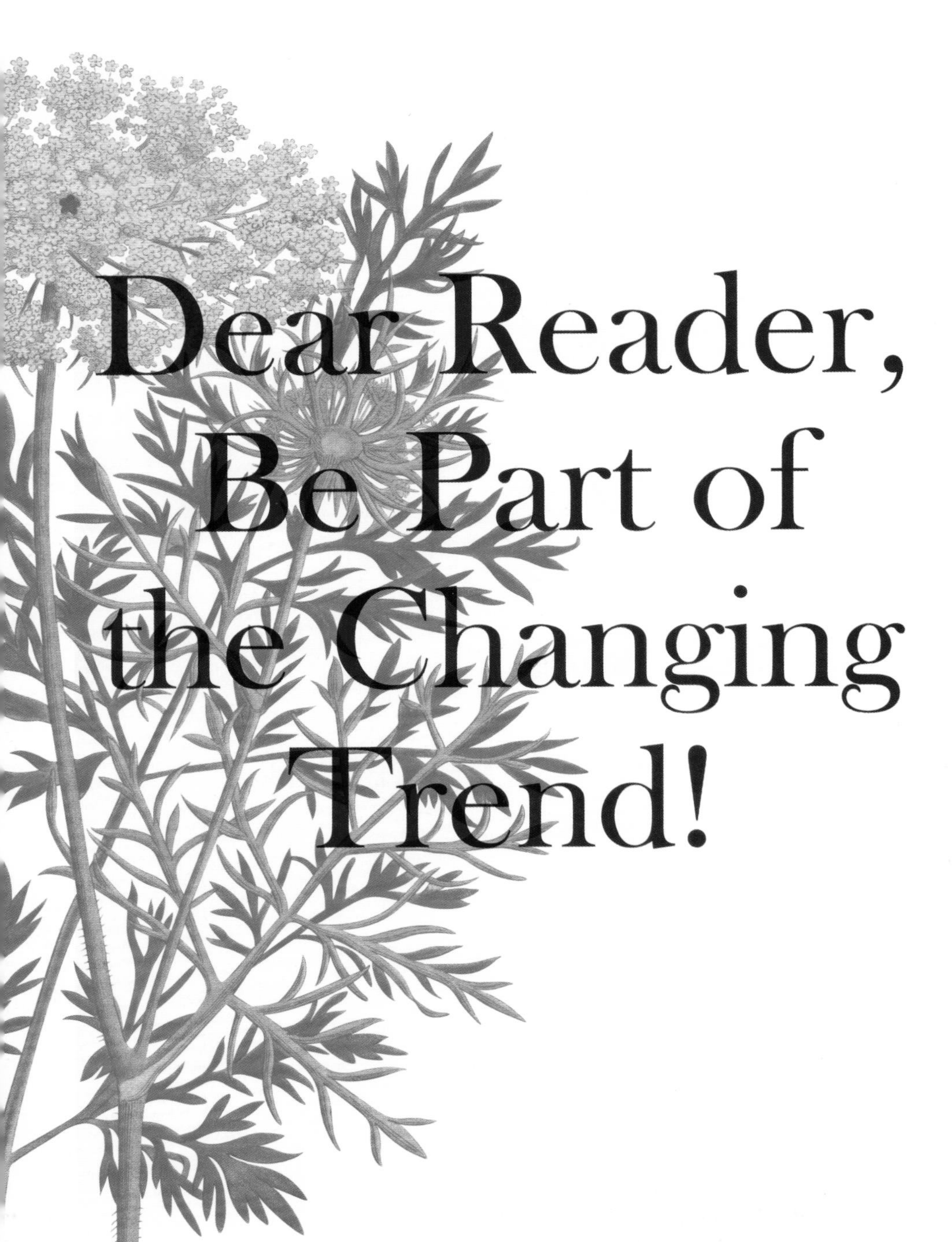

Dear Reader, Be Part of the Changing Trend!

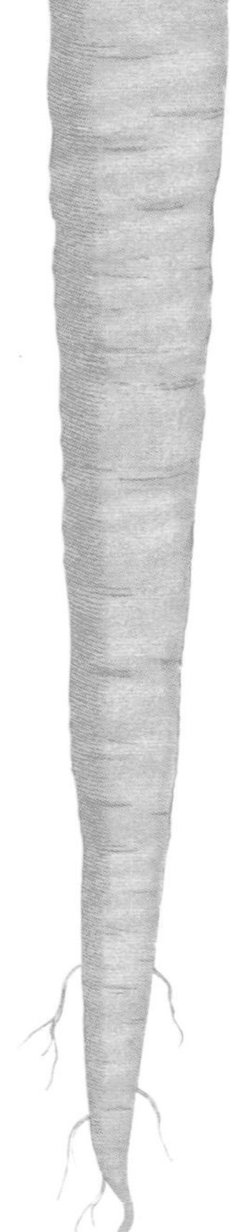

12

Perhaps you, dear reader, are already in the process of establishing a lifestyle for yourself? Possibly together with someone close, perhaps for your children?

I hope that you will receive my method in the spirit it was given: as a positive vision for the future!

And I hope that you'll adopt all the tips to make your good food habits into a pleasure.

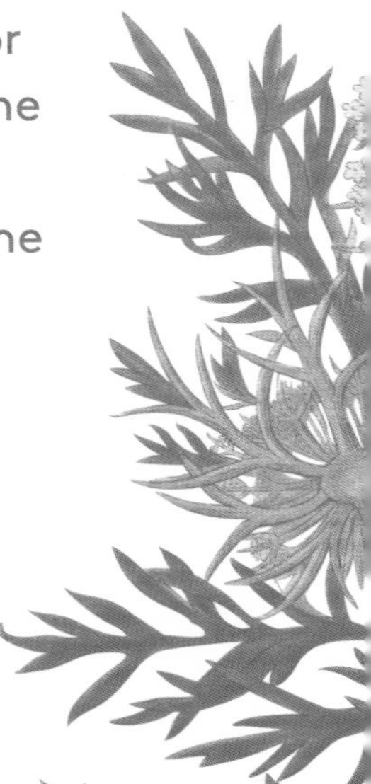

IF YOU'RE UNABLE to follow my twelve commandments for optimal health to the last letter, at least try to eat plenty of plant matter each day, and preferably raw. Minimize sugar and dairy products. Exercise regularly; it doesn't have to be strenuous. Try to protect yourself from internal stress as much as possible.

The Times Are Faring Better than the Gut

Throughout my long adult life I have most certainly seen completely different times from what you have; times that were, in many ways, actually worse. Times when dinner vegetables were a few measly boiled tinned beans along the edge of the plate. Children received sugary lollipops from aunts and uncles whenever during the school week. Work forced many out of bed at early dawn, and strict foremen oversaw the workplace. For many, exercise was just an unhurried "stretch those arms upwards." It wasn't a time when striving for a green diet, a strong body, and a harmonious interior was the easiest of tasks.

"You possess fantastic possibilities to eat yourself to better health!"

So, in other words, remember that you—in your lifetime—have fantastic possibilities to eat yourself to better health! Even the time of fast-food chains lording it as "junk food kingdom" is over. It's been quite a while now since they started selling carrots and veggie-burgers, and every diner serves unlimited raw crudités. Grocery stores also offer an increasingly larger variety of fruits and vegetables. It will be even better if we actively move to improve production methods, food handling, and food culture. Many households willingly donate their best-tasting apples in fall.

Lighted bike and exercise trails have become a given throughout Sweden. Abstaining from smoking and drinking also seems easier today than in the past when both smoking and drinking were romanticized. To exercise as needed, and to one's own ability, has perhaps become more fun when most everybody else is also running on the trail.

My hope, and my belief, is that we will learn bit by bit from our ancestors. We'll learn to see the associations among food culture, digestion, health, and movement. Increasingly, more people take an interest in the vital importance of gut health. You will be far from alone if you invest in the trend.

If You Are Expecting

For pregnant women, the choice of lifestyle is also, to an extraordinary high degree, a choice for the new individual—the child. Every expectant woman can give her child a vital advantage in life by living extra healthily during the pregnancy and the breastfeeding period and by prolonging the breastfeeding period to way past when the child has started eating solids.

Breast milk is something totally unique. A woman's milk contains namely oligosaccharides, a kind of health-giving fiber. It is something nobody has succeeded in reproducing synthetically, and the same form does not exist in the milk of other species. In addition, there are specific lactobacilli in the milk the child readily accepts and carries the rest of their life.

STRIKE AGAINST OVERINDULGENCE— FOR THE CHILD'S SAKE

We have mentioned earlier how Europeans and Americans in the middle of the twentieth century started to dramatically change our food habits and turn to processed foods. This development is very difficult to resist for expectant mothers—but it is vital for the sake of the child.

The truth is, today's mothers are getting more and more overweight and giving birth to bigger and bigger babies. Gunnar Meeuwisse, a pediatrician, once told me that during the last hundred years we've had to revise upward the "normal" (i.e., the average) birth weight no fewer than four times. It is reported that the number of overweight expectant women in delivery rooms in Sweden at the end of the twentieth century doubled in just ten years. It continues to increase at the same speed.

YOUR BODY WEIGHT AND HEALTH HAVE BIG REPERCUSSIONS FOR YOUR CHILD

The recommended weight gain during pregnancy ought to stay below thirty-three pounds (15 kg), and preferably lower.

Nearly 75 percent of obese women blame pregnancy as the triggering factor for their later permanent overweight condition. Many also seem to use the pregnancy as an excuse to eat much more than usual; "eating for two" is a commonly heard expression.

> "If you choose to follow my method, just put my commandments for optimal health on your refrigerator door and follow them as best as you can."

In Great Britain and North America (and very probably also in South America) it's not uncommon for many new babies' birth weights to be between 17½ to 22 pounds (8–10 kg). It is a well-known fact that overweight pregnant women have a high level of inflammation. Their broken-down gut flora results in an inferior immune system and slow metabolism. The inflammatory burden in the mother also stresses the unborn child.

Women with high BMI also have an increased need for cesarean sections. Complication frequency is increased for these women during surgical as well as normal births.

Anything that disturbs the process during pregnancy and breast-feeding—such as excessive hygiene, wrong diet, artificial formula, pharmaceuticals (especially antibiotics during foster and neonatal period and the early childhood years)—plays an important role in future health.

It really isn't just a question of abstaining from alcohol and tobacco. Considerably more efforts are demanded for optimal results. If you choose to follow my method, just put my commandments for optimal health on your refrigerator door and follow them as best as you can.

STRONG ASSOCIATIONS BETWEEN UTERINE ENVIRONMENT AND CHRONIC ILLNESS

It was the British professor of pediatrics David J. P. Barker who at the beginning of 1900 observed that chronic illness in later life doesn't just happen through a combination of adult lifestyle and genetics. He also found that the uterine environment and the mother's body played an important role. He reported that even short periods of stress on the unborn in the uterus could lead to permanent changes/impairment/reprogramming of the child's immune system and lead to permanent changes in blood pressure, cholesterol metabolism, insulin response to sugar, and a list of metabolic, endocrine, and immune parameters.

Later studies have confirmed Barker's observations. It is also calculated that the influence during pregnancy is about 30 percent, while about 70 percent is dependent on the individual's adult lifestyle. I also want to mention a recent Norwegian study that shows important observations. It describes how children of high birth weight have a tendency to develop immune diseases such as type 1 diabetes at double the rate of babies of normal birth weight.

The factors contributing to increased allergies, in the mother's lifestyle before and during the pregnancy and breastfeeding period, include exposure to endotoxins (dust in the air and unsuitable foods), tobacco, contamination and environmental toxins, climate changes, and many more. We're often talking about the same elements that have shown themselves to contribute to chronic illnesses later in life. The difference is, during pregnancy you don't only affect your own susceptibility but also that of the child.

LACTOBACILLUS SHOWED POSITIVE RESULTS

The Finnish researchers Erika Isolauri and Seppo Salminen and their colleagues released a study in 2003 showing how adding lactobacillus to the mother during her last months of pregnancy and to the child during its first six months, could nearly halve the frequency of allergy occurrence in children. This applied to children born into especially allergy-prone families.

They returned with a new study when the children reached puberty and it actually showed that with this treatment they had managed to completely stave off both ADHD and Asperger's syndrome, while 17 percent of the children who did not have access to this treatment developed both these diseases.

I have worked with my synbiotics for many years and know well their fantastic anti-inflammatory properties. I wish that all expectant mothers could get access to synbiotics, at least during the last months of their pregnancy and the child's first months. The mothers lubricating the nipples with synbiotics both before and after breastfeeding can do this.

Decide. And Dare!

Finally, let me declare forcefully:

It really isn't just up to expectant women to take on all the responsibility for the lifestyle they choose. In many instances there is a partner who can affect, ease, and profoundly share the responsibility.

Yes, you're all part of a whole—every one of my readers—where your own food habits and health principles may have a large impact on others.

My belief is that you, as an individual, can get many to accompany you if you decide on a life based on the Anti-Inflammatory Diet Solution's ideas.

It is all about deciding to do it, and then to dare.

Someone who dared was former president Bill Clinton. He was an extreme "junk-food addict" and could have his ten-car motorcade stop in front of McDonald's to get the day's hamburger and

French fries. He eventually developed a serious heart condition, probably partly stress-induced, and because of a lack of proper exercise. His physician, Dean Ornish, gave him an ultimatum: "Follow my health regimen to 100 percent." The program contained—sounds familiar?—plenty of raw food, stress control, very small amounts of cooking oils, exercise, and a rich social life.

Ornish knew that every reduced percentage point of cholesterol improves the chance for a healthy life. We who think along these lines have long taken an interest in whether vitamin K2 can have a central part in a development like Clinton's. Because of new observations, this question has awakened a new interest in me. One of my new goals is to investigate just this!

So how did it go for Clinton? Well, he regained his health and has lived since 2011 like a true health zealot!

So, decide to get yourself a food processor and a spiralizer. Make the children bright red or green and white clouds of spaghetti strands from raw red beets and zucchini. Start a smoothie culture at home—use flash-frozen fruits and berries, in large beautiful glasses, with thick fun straws. Go ahead and learn tasty new recipes that don't require a lot of butter, fat, or cooking. Get used to cold food—it is after all no fun to clean saucepans.

Throw out everything left behind in the pantry that feels aged and unwholesome.

Dare to throw children's parties that won't descend into orgies of whipped cream and sugar. Other parents will love you for it, and your children will be proud.

Dare to stop eating before you're full.

Dare try intermittent fasting. (Teenagers have long practiced this by sleeping until midday.)

Perhaps you have an opportunity to work for better health consciousness at work or in your community?

Fresh dietary habits will make your body stronger, that's for certain. It becomes more fun to exercise. All of a sudden, you will sit down, just for the pleasure of it, on a tree stump in the woods and just relax and feel good.

Recipes

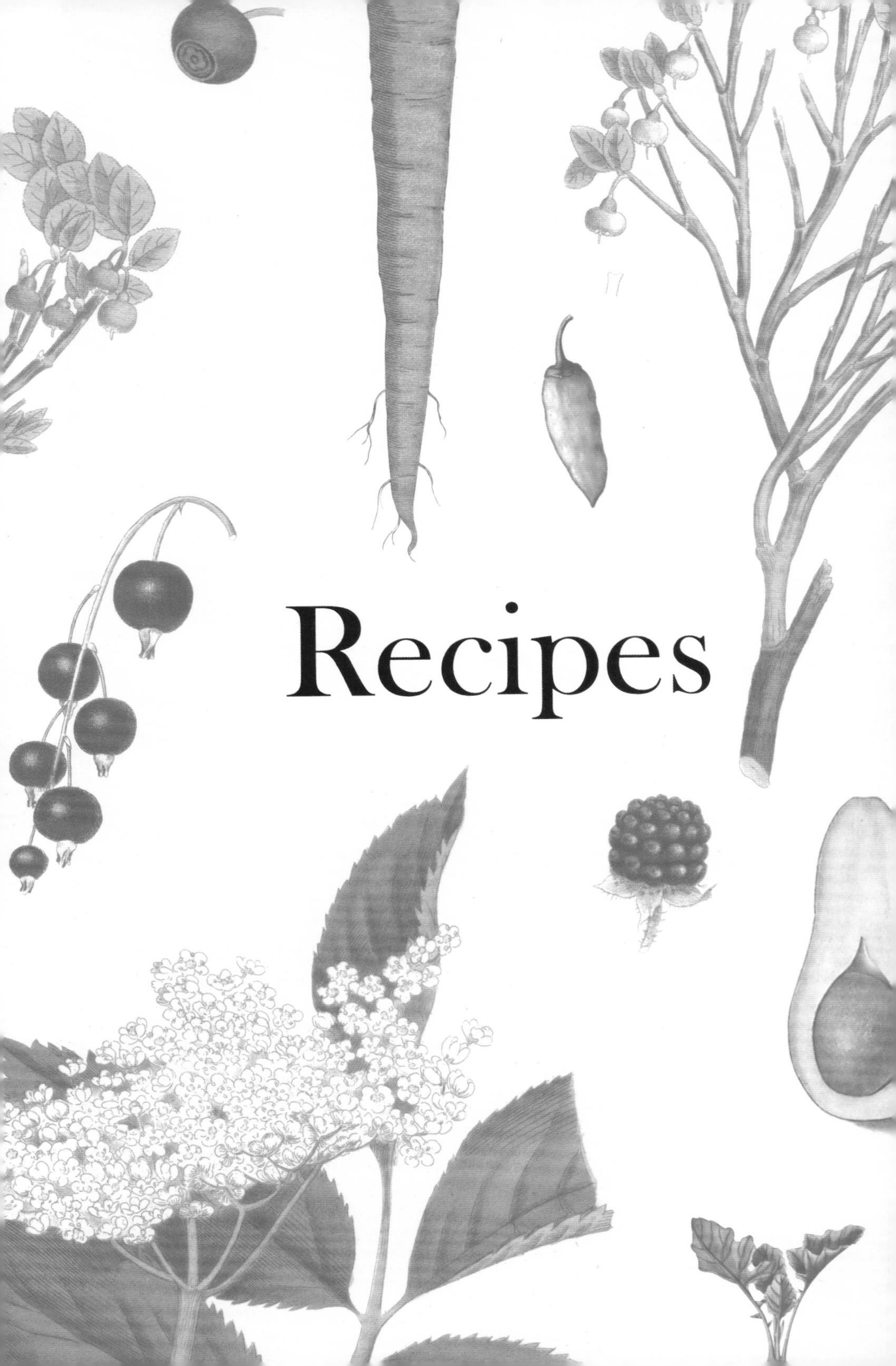

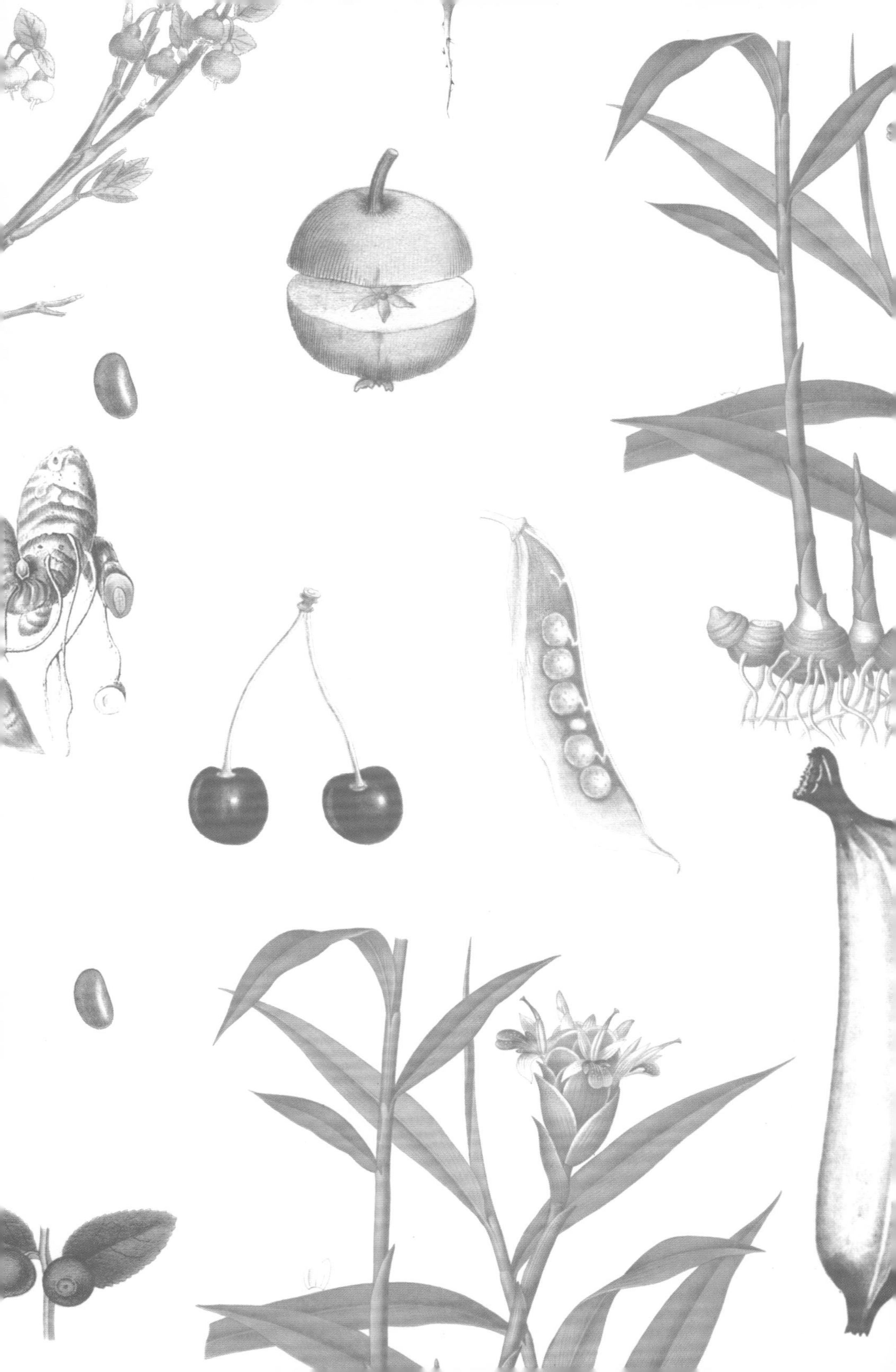

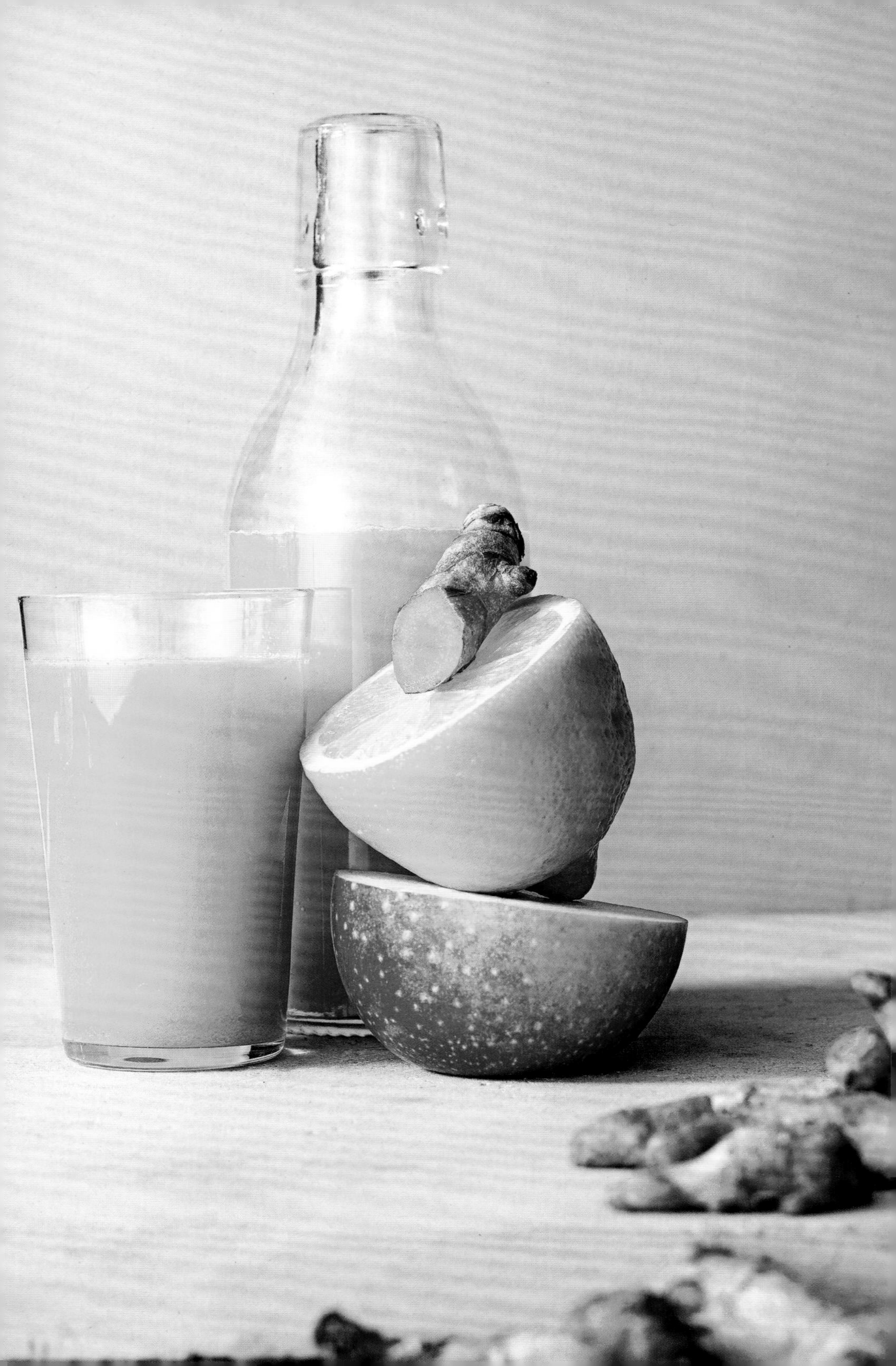

Stig's Anti-Inflammatory Turmeric Cocktail

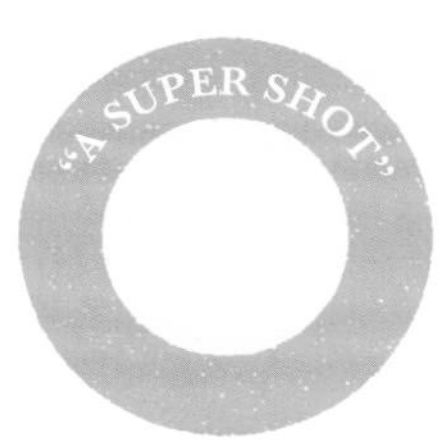

SERVES 1

½ glass or 1 glass fruit juice (pineapple, apple, or similar)
1 heaping tablespoon ground turmeric
Approx. ¼ teaspoon cayenne pepper (don't exceed)
¾ tablespoon (1 dessert spoon) ground Ceylon cinnamon
1 teaspoon cumin
Small pinch ground cloves
½ teaspoon–1 tablespoon apple cider vinegar
1 teaspoon lemon juice

Mix all the ingredients and drink once or twice a day. An alternative is to get fresh turmeric and dice it finely and mix into the daily salad.

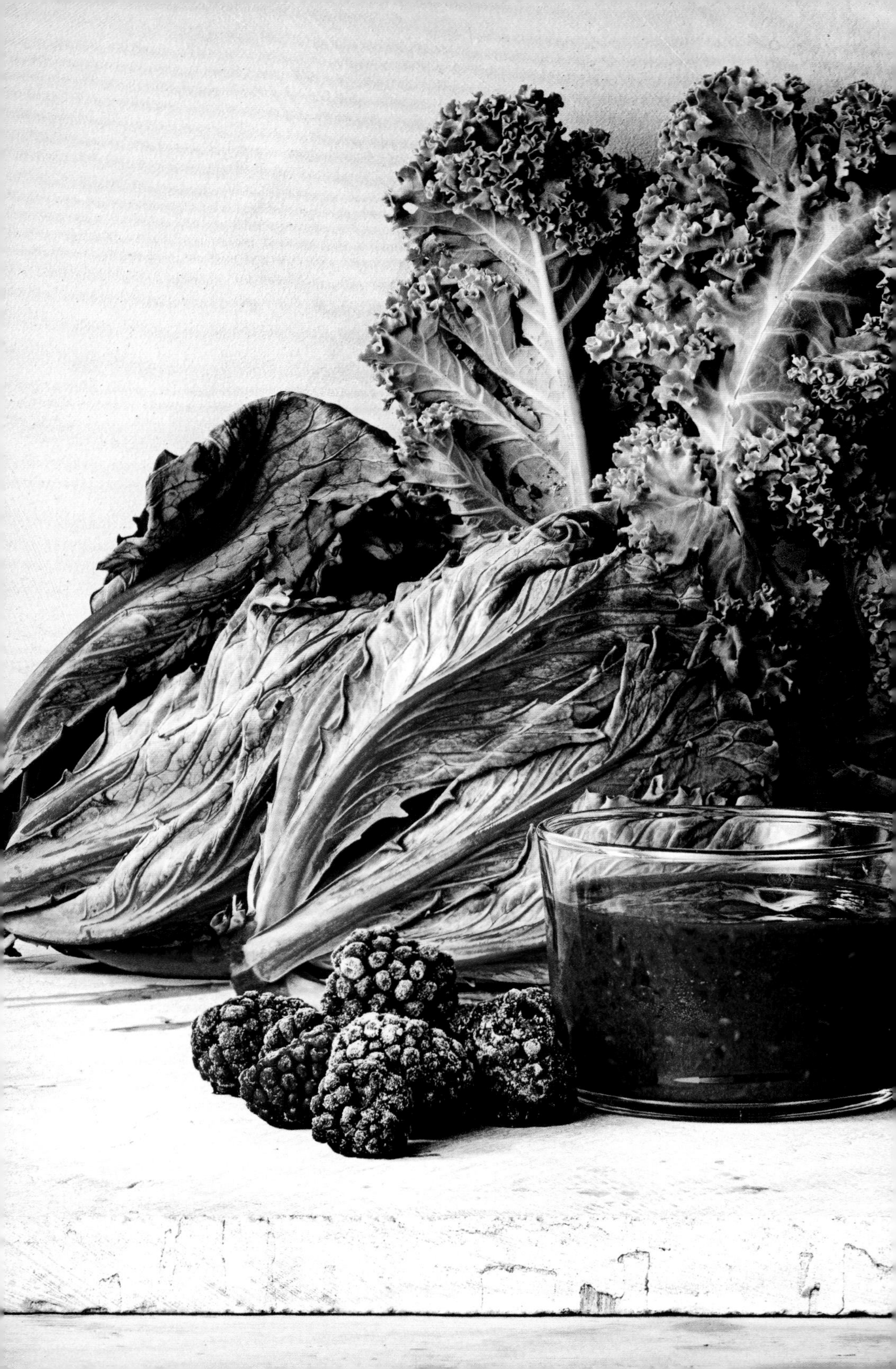

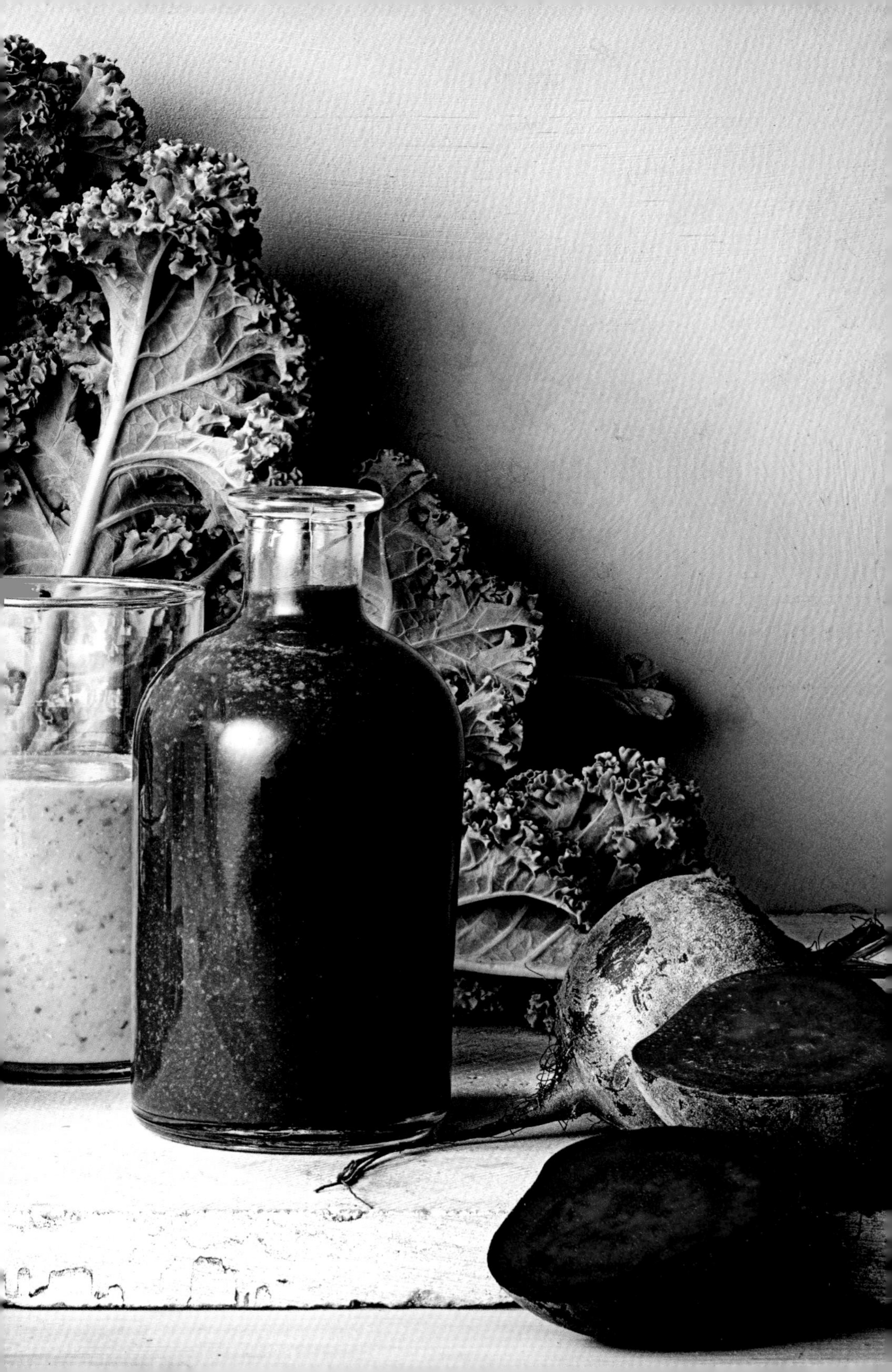

Smoothie—Basic Recipe

4 ¼ cups (1 liter) water
Mix of root vegetables such as raw potatoes, carrots with tops, beets with tops, other leafy greens, avocado, and celery
Some fruits, for ex. unpeeled apple with core or a kiwi
Piece of fresh ginger, garlic, or onion
¼–1 lime or lemon with peel
1 tablespoon psyllium husk
1 heaping tablespoon ground turmeric
½–1 tablespoon spirulina
½ tablespoon coconut oil

Always add heart-healthy turmeric and avocado, both for goodness and creaminess. Then vary with what takes your fancy. No need to add garlic if you don't like it. Double the ginger if you like the taste! That root is brimming with antioxidants.

(Marianne and I usually bring grated ginger and turmeric on our travels.)

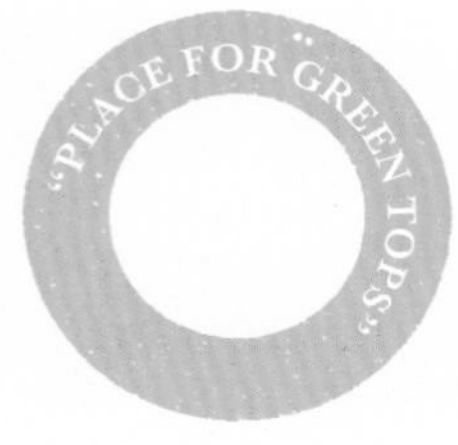

Smoothie with Beet Greens

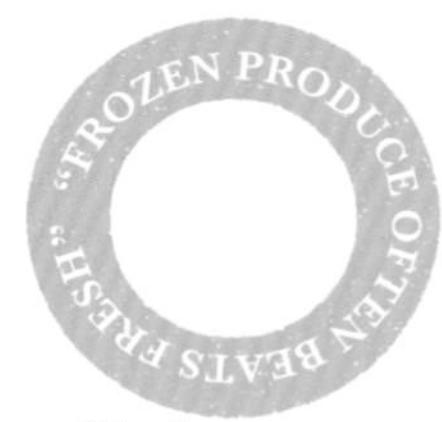

2⅛ cups (½ liter) mixed berries (here it's good to go with frozen raspberries, blackberries, or strawberries)
Hint agave syrup
6–8 beet greens and stalks
Extra water to dilute the smoothie if needed

Here you make several good choices. Flash-frozen berries usually retain many more nutrients than fresh berries that have had extensive handling.

Remember that the beet greens and stalks contain much less sugar than the beet itself. The greens also contain lots of beneficial magnesium.

Marianne's Super Healthy Green Beverage

½ pound (250 g) kale
1 cup (2 dl) rolled oats
4¼ cups (1 liter) water
2 avocados
1 apple
⅕ teaspoon (1 krm) grated nutmeg
1 tsp. iodized salt or Seltin [Swedish mineral salt]
⅕ teaspoon (1 krm) ground white pepper
1–2 teaspoon chervil

Mix it all and pour into a large pitcher.

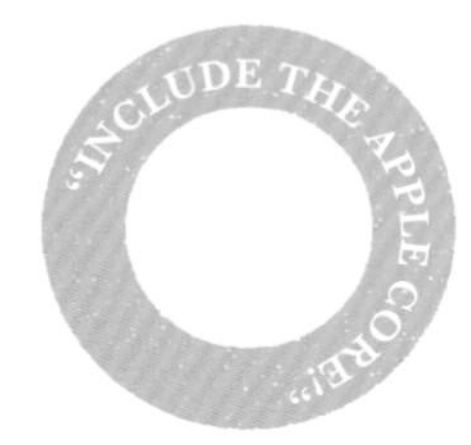

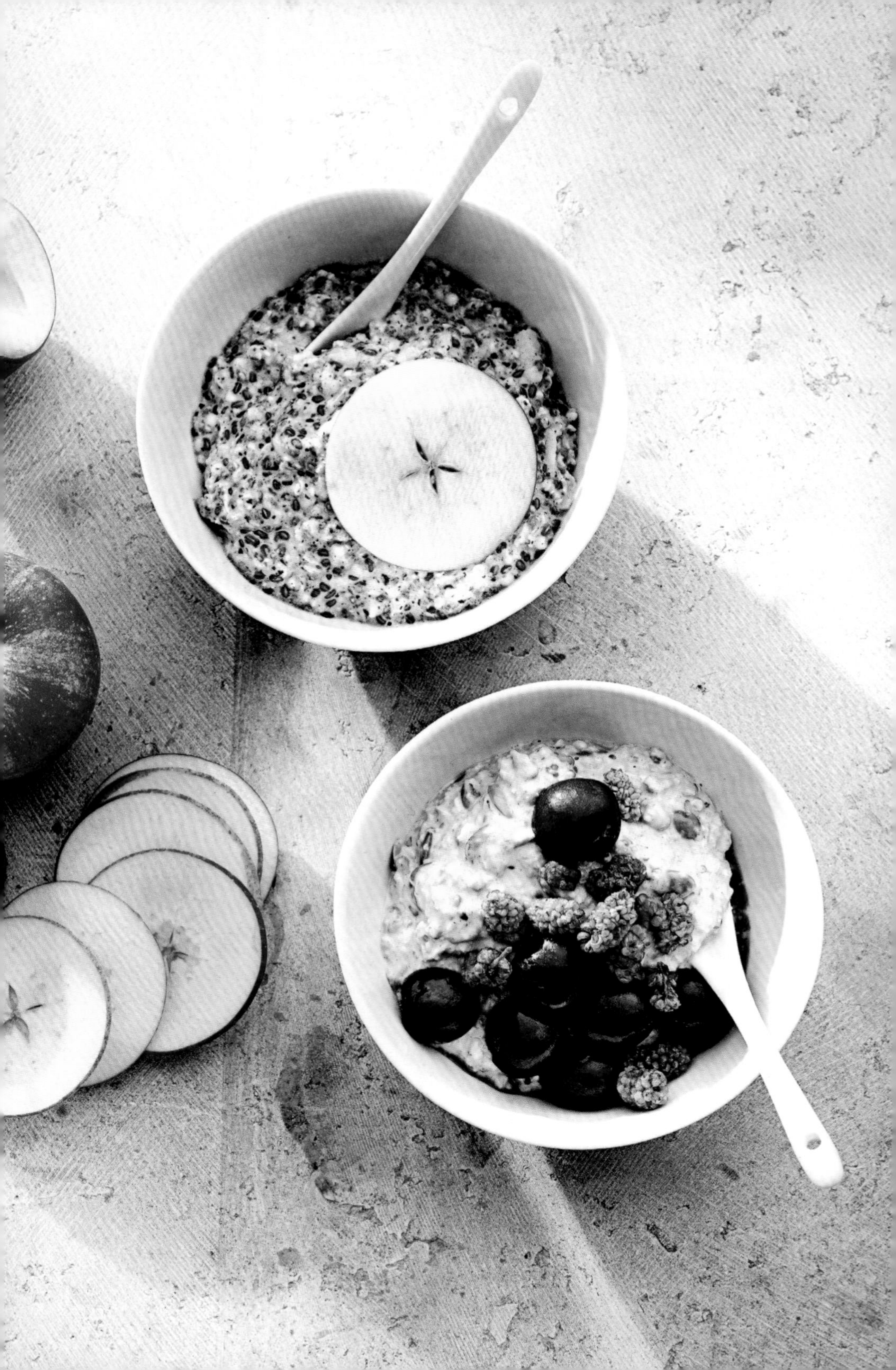

Bircher Muesli

2 tablespoons pumpkin seeds
2 tablespoons sunflower seeds
⅔ cup (1½ dl) rolled oats
1 tablespoon hemp hearts
1 tablespoon mulberries
3 tablespoons coconut yogurt
½ cup (1 dl) almond or other vegetable beverage, unsweetened
⅔ cup (1½ dl) cherries or other fruit

Our version here of the original well-known Bircher muesli is often called overnight oats. Cut the cherries and mulberries in half if you prefer them that way. They contain a wealth of seeds that become extra nutritious and bioavailable for the body if you soak them in the jar overnight. It's a pleasure to wake up to a ready-made muesli mix! The muesli got its name after Maximilian Bircher-Brenner, a Swiss physician who introduced it to his patients at the sanatorium in Zürichberg. It was served as a light evening meal and contained grated apple, rolled oats, nuts, and milk—and lemon to protect the apple from discoloration.

"OVERNIGHT OATS"

Our Own Bircher Muesli

1 cup (2 dl) rolled oats
2 tablespoons psyllium husks (soak for 24 hours in a separate bowl)
2 tablespoons sumac
½ cup (½ dl) durrah
2 tablespoons chia seeds
1 grated apple
Grated Ceylon cinnamon, to taste
1½–2 cups (3–4 dl) water

Marianne's and my interest in trying out nutritious novelties made us add both the spice sumac—an umami taste with a touch of lemon—and the popular African grain durrah. Very pleasing result! Preparation can start the night before: soak the psyllium husks in a separate bowl for twenty-four hours—it's well worth the effort. Imagine the amount of nutritious seed and peel we've usually given up and only fed to our animals.

"TIME FOR SUMAC"

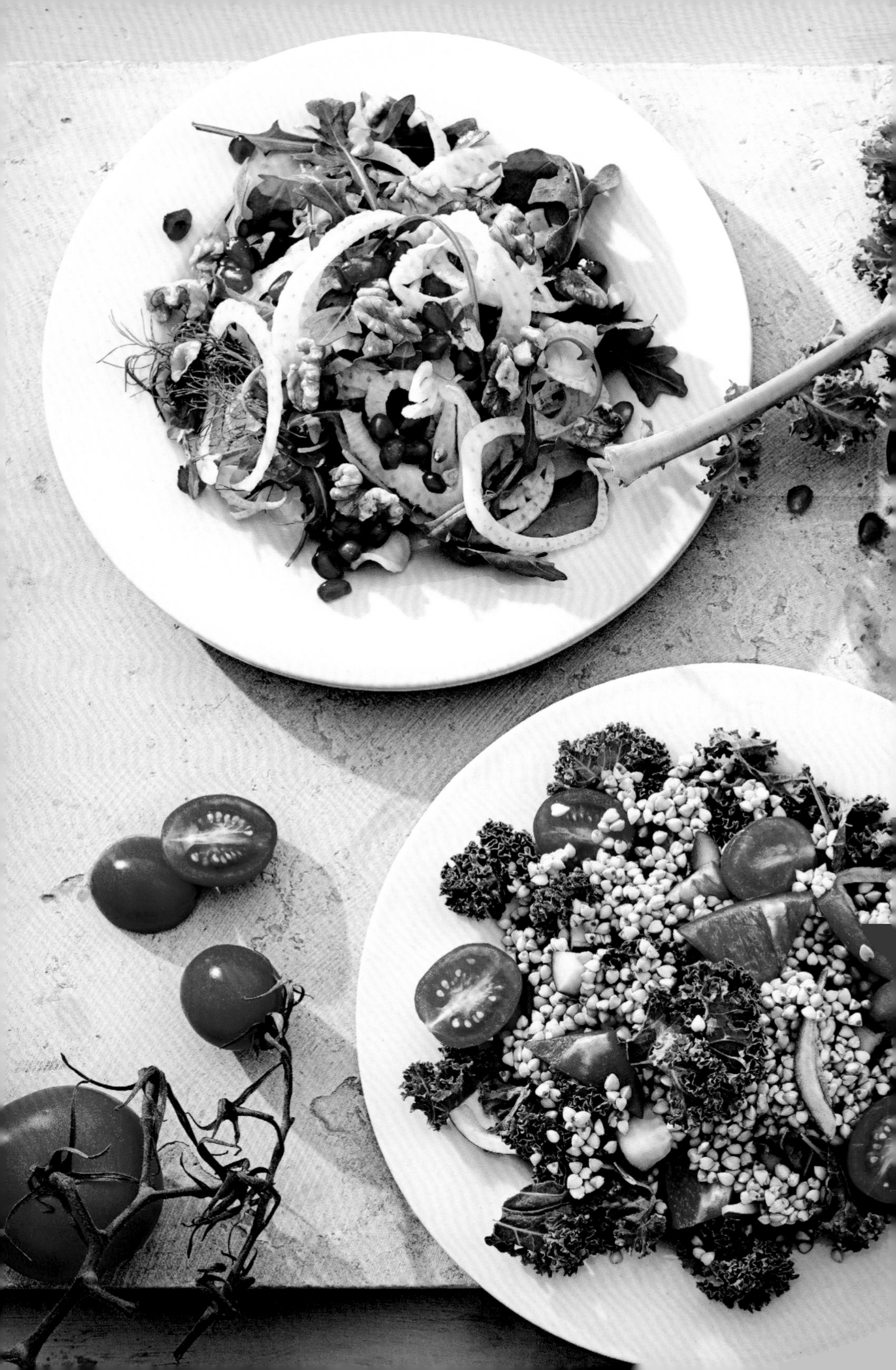

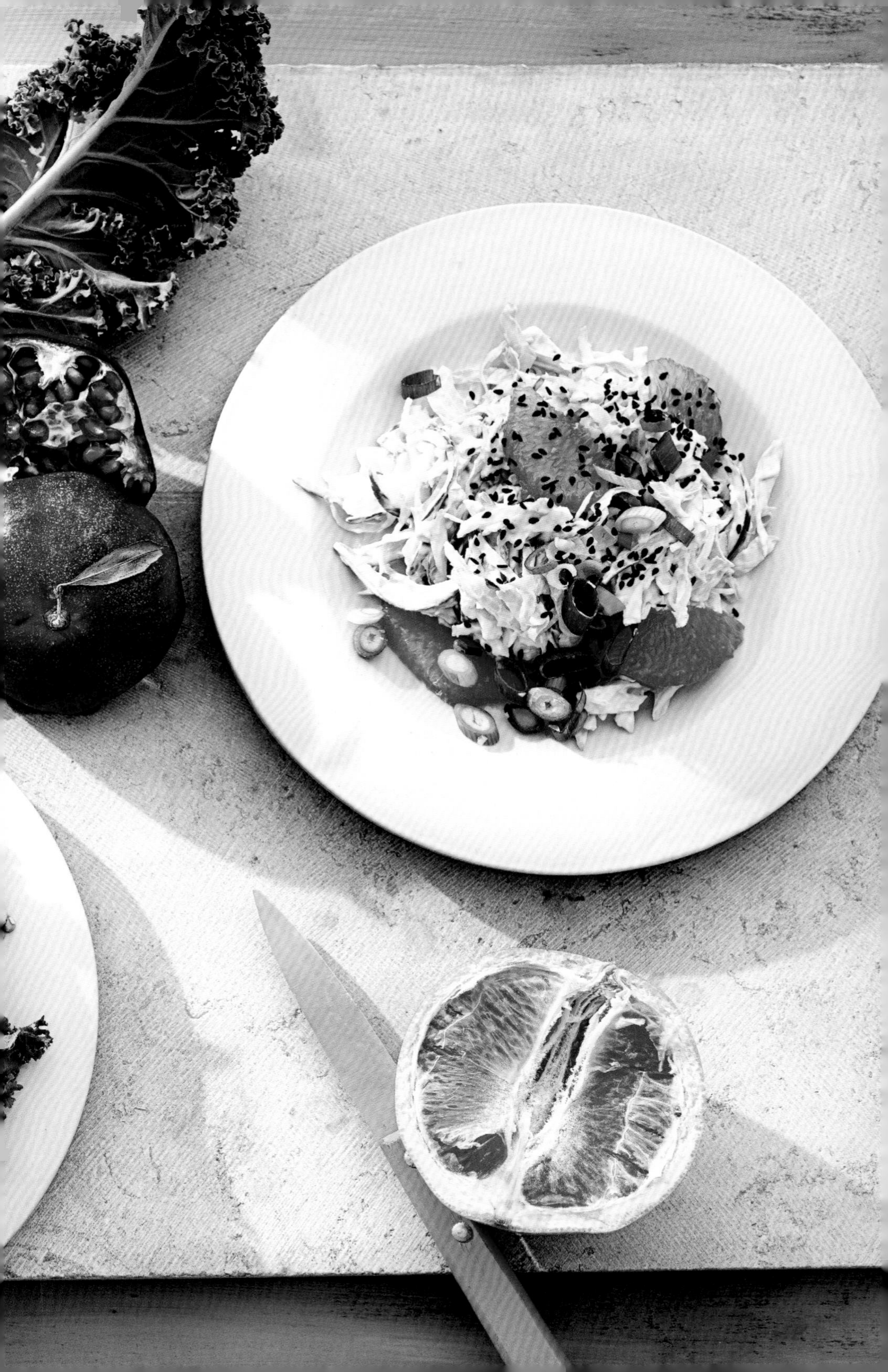

Fennel Salad

½ head fennel, shaved very thinly
½ bunch arugula
½ pomegranate
5 walnuts, chopped coarsely

This is a delicious salad with beautiful colors and unique flavors. Mix the fennel and arugula with the pomegranate seeds. It's best to use a kitchen mandolin for the fennel to get superthin slices! Exquisite. Sprinkle with chopped walnuts.

"SUPERTHIN SLICES"

Marianne's Buckwheat Sprinkled Kale Salad

SERVES 4
½ small red onion
3 tablespoons apple cider vinegar
6 tablespoons coconut oil
1 pound (500 g) kale
½ pound (250 g) buckwheat
½ pound (¼ kg) cherry tomatoes, quartered
¼ cucumber, cut into matchsticks
1 red bell pepper, cut into matchsticks
Iodized salt
Freshly ground pepper

Soak the buckwheat for eight hours in advance if you use it raw. If cooking, follow the instructions on the packaging.

Grate the (steamed or raw) kale into smaller pieces in a bowl. Add the chopped onion, cherry tomatoes, cucumber, and bell pepper, coconut oil, and vinegar. Mix. Sprinkle the salad with the buckwheat—raw, warm, or cooked and then cooled. Season with salt and pepper.

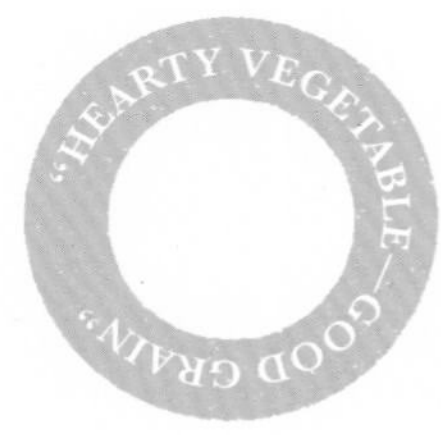

Raw Coleslaw

1 small head white cabbage
1 red onion
1 cup (2 dl) nondairy crème fraîche
1 teaspoon Dijon mustard
1 tablespoon coconut oil
1 tablespoon lemon juice
Iodized salt
Freshly ground black pepper

DRESSINGS

MUSTARD AND VINEGAR

1 cup (2 dl) grated carrot
1 teaspoon French mustard
½ teaspoon white wine vinegar

TAHINI AND GINGER

1 grated carrot
2 teaspoons tahini
1½ tablespoons grated fresh ginger
Zest and juice of 1 lime
2 teaspoons honey
¼–½ cup (½–1 dl) fresh mint

GRAPE AND SRIRACHA

2 grapefruits in segments, pith removed
2 teaspoons chili sauce
2 salad onions, sliced finely
1 tablespoon black or white sesame seeds

Shred the white cabbage and red onion. Mix the rest of the ingredients and add to the cabbage and onion. For best results, let the salad rest overnight. Serve this with diced apple and/or with one of the suggested dressings.

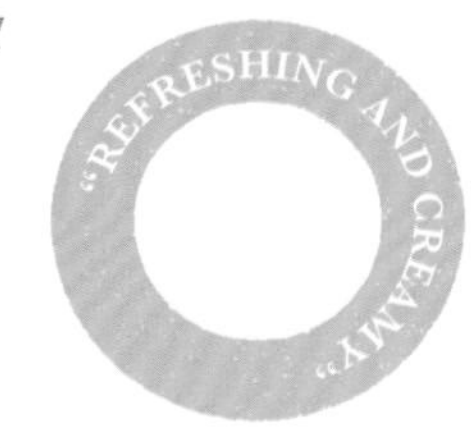

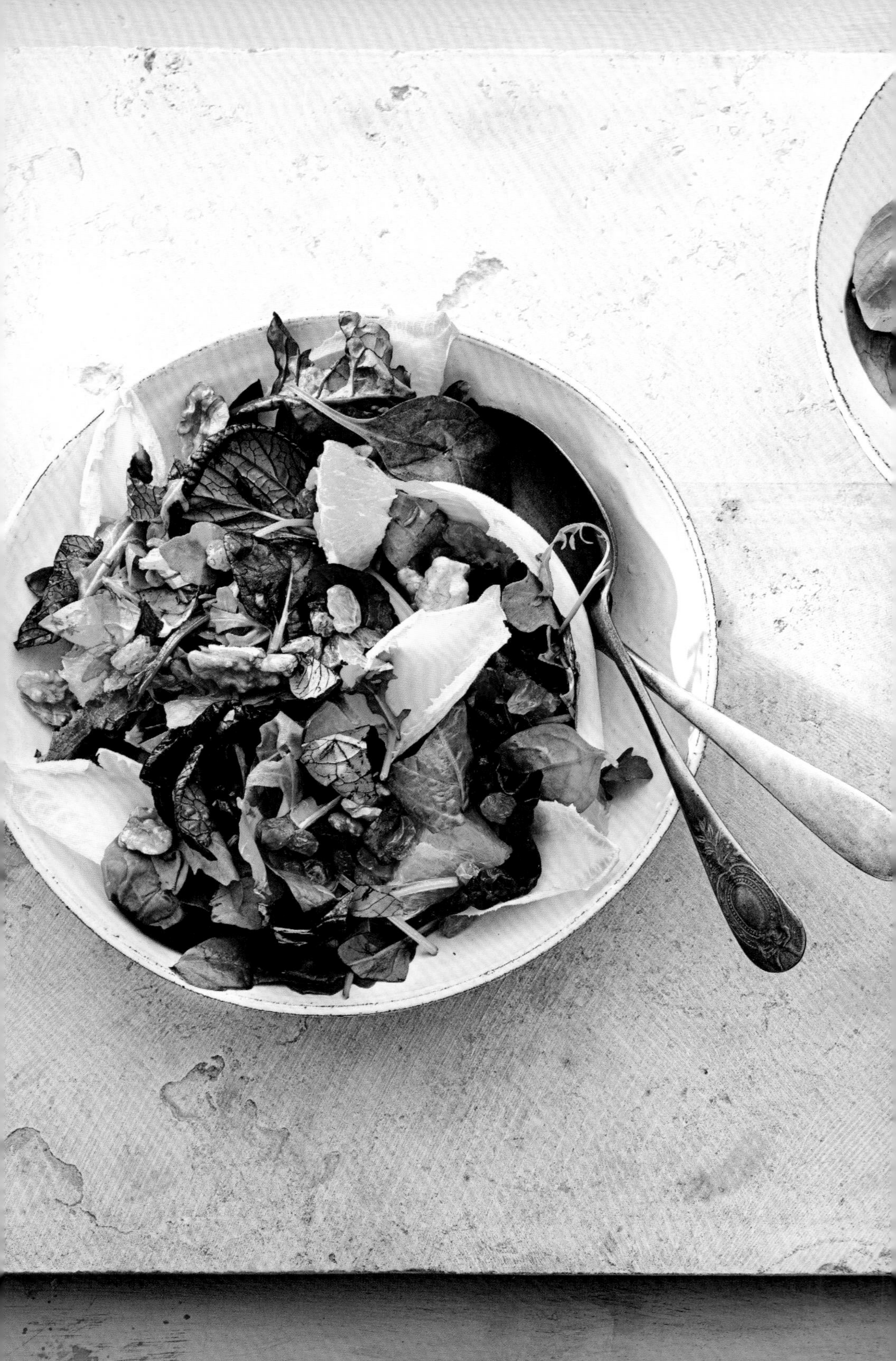

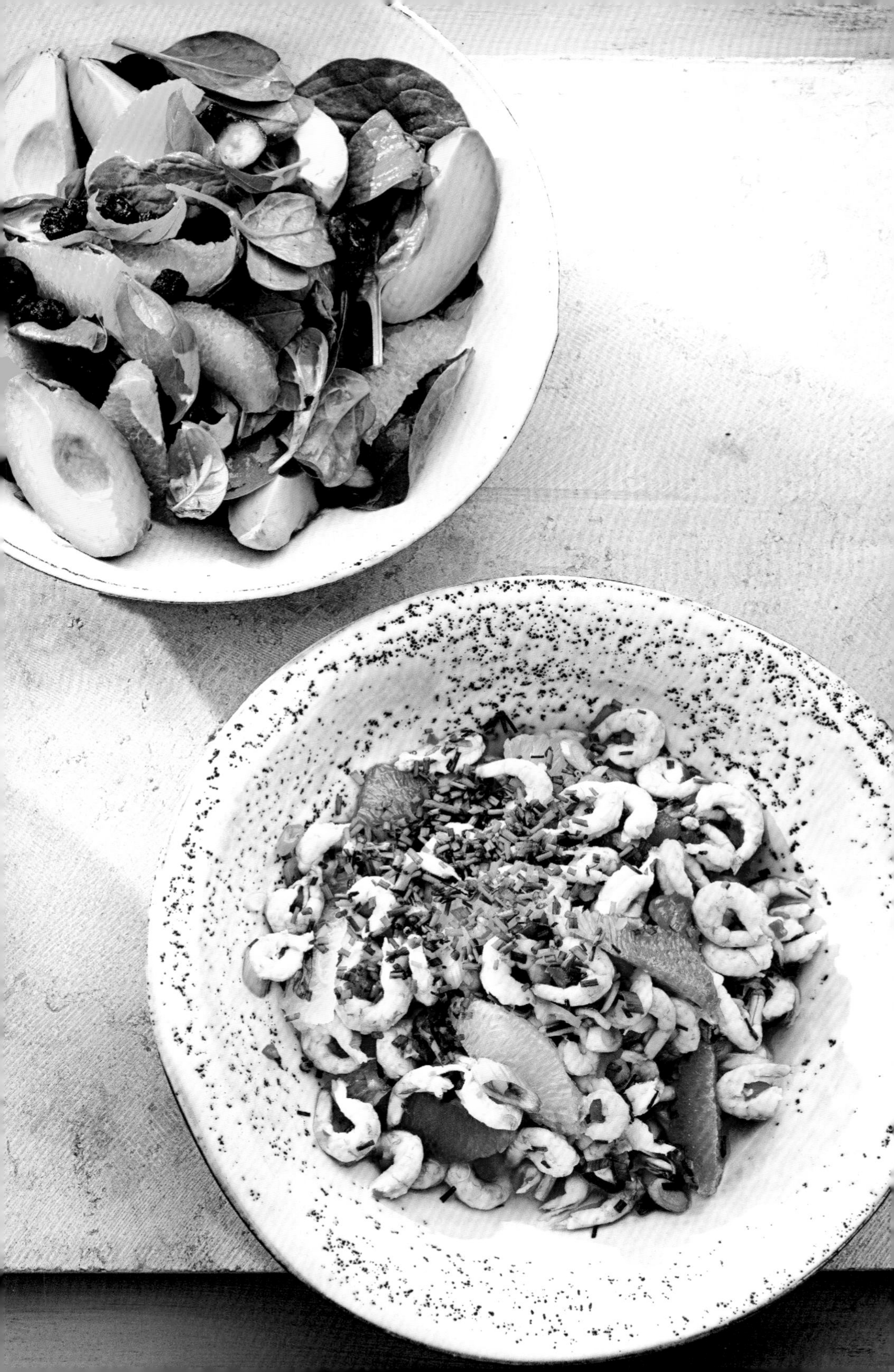

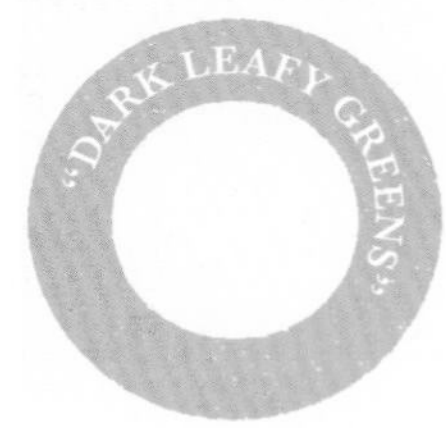

Endive with Mixed Leafy Greens

SERVES 4
1 pound (500 g) mixed leafy greens
1 grapefruit
2 oranges
1 or 2 endives
1 cup (2 dl) cranberries
½ cup (1 dl) walnuts

DRESSING
2 tablespoons orange juice, freshly juiced
3 tablespoons coconut oil
2 tablespoons water
Iodized salt, pepper, and herbs if so desired

Pick over a selection of dark-colored leafy greens; they are bursting with goodness! Choose according to your preference, for example, arugula, chard, and broccoli. Arugula contains the good MCT (medium-chain triglycerides), and broccoli is relatively free of pesticide residue.

Shred the leaves coarsely. Measure out about 1½–2 cups (3–4 dl) of shredded greens. Peel the grapefruit and the oranges. Dice them or remove the pith and use whole segments. Mix salad greens and citrus fruit. Mix the ingredients for the dressing, pour over the salad, and mix.

Arrange the salad on a platter. Separate the endive leaves and garnish the salad with them. Coarsely chop the walnuts and sprinkle nuts and cranberries over the salad.

Spinach Salad with Blueberries and Almonds

“NOTE! POTENT SPRINKLES!”

SERVES 2
10½ ounces (300 g) spinach
Diced flesh of 1 ripe avocado
1 fresh basil plant, shredded
1 orange, peeled and diced or segmented, pith removed

TO SERVE
½ cup (1 dl) bilberries
½ cup (1 dl) almonds
¼ cup (½ dl) tahini dressing

The spinach can be replaced with kale or mixed with arugula and chard. Tear the leafy greens into approx. 2-inch x 2-inch (5 cm x 5 cm) pieces. Why not add your favorite sprouts and shoots, too? Rinse everything in cold water first, and then let dry thoroughly. In a bowl, mix the ingredients with the dressing, then massage the dressing into the salad.

Carefully fold in the avocado, basil, and orange. Arrange this on the plates. Sprinkle over the antioxidant-rich bilberries and almonds. They are rich in vegetable protein and omega-3. Serve the salad with the tahini dressing seasoned with sesame seeds and lemon juice.

Grapefruit and Shrimp Salad

SERVES 4

¾ pound (400 g) wild-caught tiger (scampi) or usual shrimp, cooked and peeled
1 teaspoon honey
2 tablespoons fish sauce
4 chili peppers, seeded and finely chopped
4 grapefruits, peeled and pith removed from segments
1 tablespoon freshly squeezed lime juice
3–4 salad onions, thinly sliced
Iodized salt or Seltin

GARNISH

Season with freshly chopped chives or other fresh herbs

Bring water to boil in a saucepan and cook the raw shrimp until red and firm, approximately 2 minutes. Drain off the water and put the shrimp to the side.

In the still-warm saucepan, mix the honey, fish sauce, and chili. Add the grapefruit, lime juice, onion, and shrimp. Season with salt, as organic tiger shrimps aren't salted.

Arrange the mixture on a platter and garnish with chopped chives.

We happily counteract the grapefruit's bitterness with some sweetness in a beverage. A semidry Riesling works very well here. Or perhaps choose a lighter, somewhat toffee-like and fruity ale.

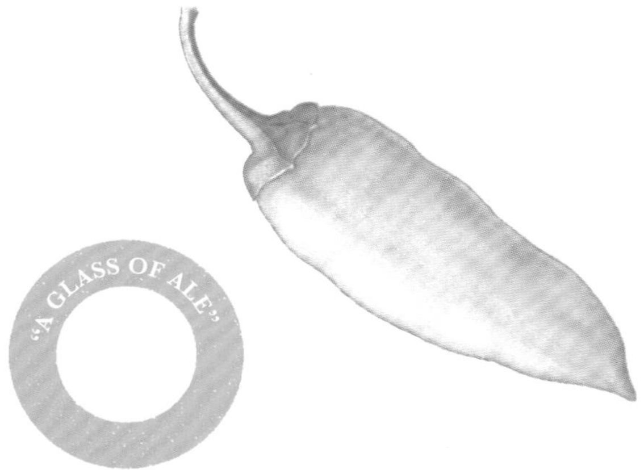

The Cloud Factory

SERVES 4 TO 6

1 large zucchini
1 bunch beets
10 large carrots
1 daikon radish
2 white spring turnips
. . . and whatever else takes your fancy in the fresh vegetable aisle

Are the children turning their noses up at raw vegetables? Not so surprising if it is the same thing day in and day out (it gets old with those cucumber slices and the pile of grated carrots).

Turn the kitchen into a cloud factory! Let the spiralizer and slicing attachments show what they can do. The kids will soon beat you at crafting thin vegetable strands into lots of "spaghetti clouds"! Except, of course, the daikon radish and the spring turnips, which have to be shaved into transparent slices that are then stuck into the vegetable clouds.

Sprinkle the whole with pea shoots, seed, and nuts as you see fit. Why not serve it all with Super Healthy Mayonnaise?

Super Healthy Mayonnaise

1 egg yolk, preferably from free-range poultry
1 teaspoon apple cider vinegar
1 teaspoon Dijon mustard
½ cup (1 dl) coconut oil
Iodized salt
Freshly ground black pepper
Garlic, chili, or similar seasonings, optional

Mix the yolk with salt; add vinegar and mustard. Make sure the bowl and all ingredients are at room temperature. Carefully add the oil drop by drop while whisking vigorously until the mixture starts to look like mayonnaise. Season with salt and pepper. Add garlic, fresh chili, and favorite spices if you so desire.

Make the mayonnaise greener and heartier by mixing in, at the end, finely chopped raw asparagus, fennel, or other non-waterlogged vegetables.

"OK, GO AHEAD, USE AN EGG YOLK"

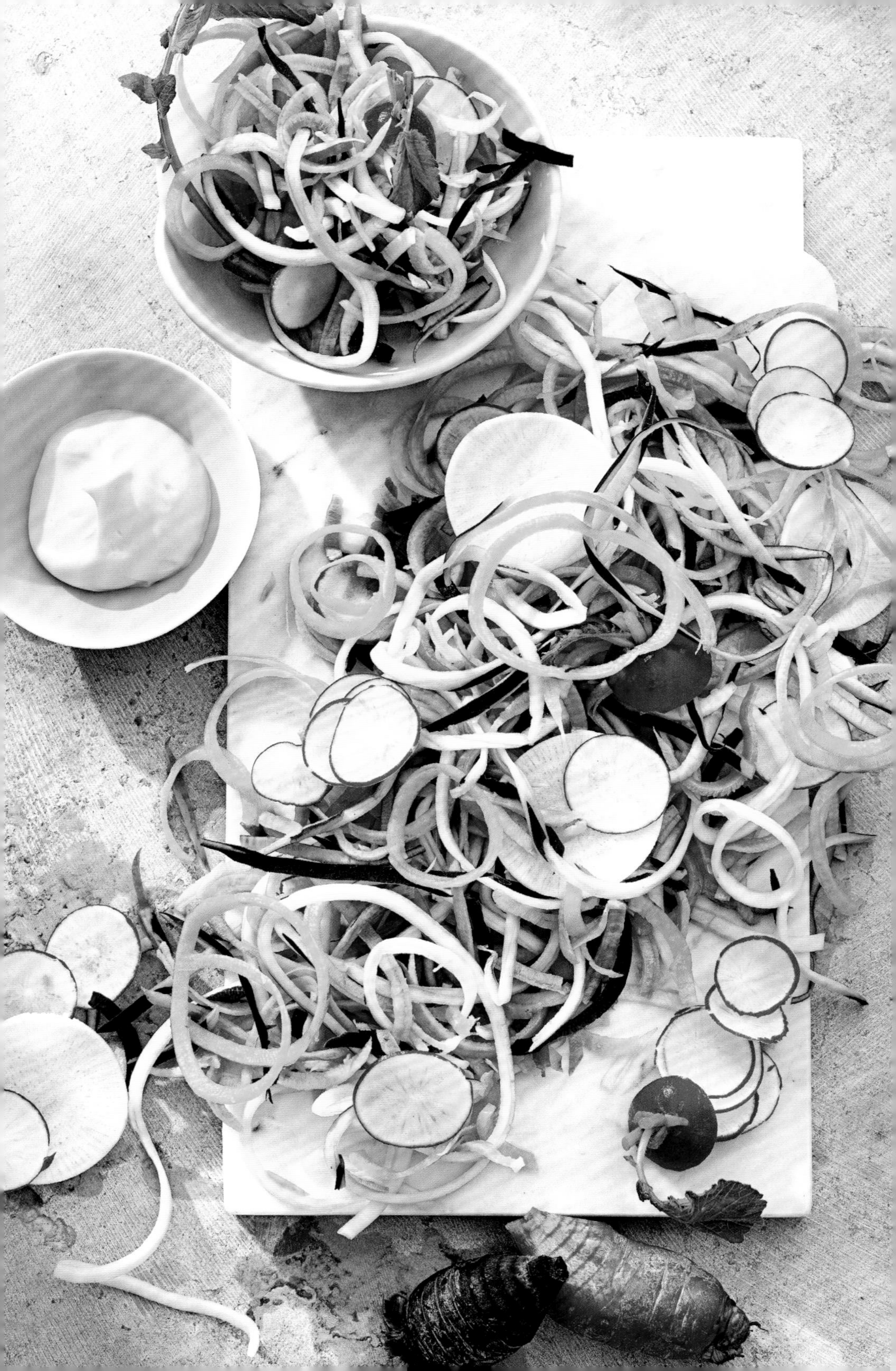

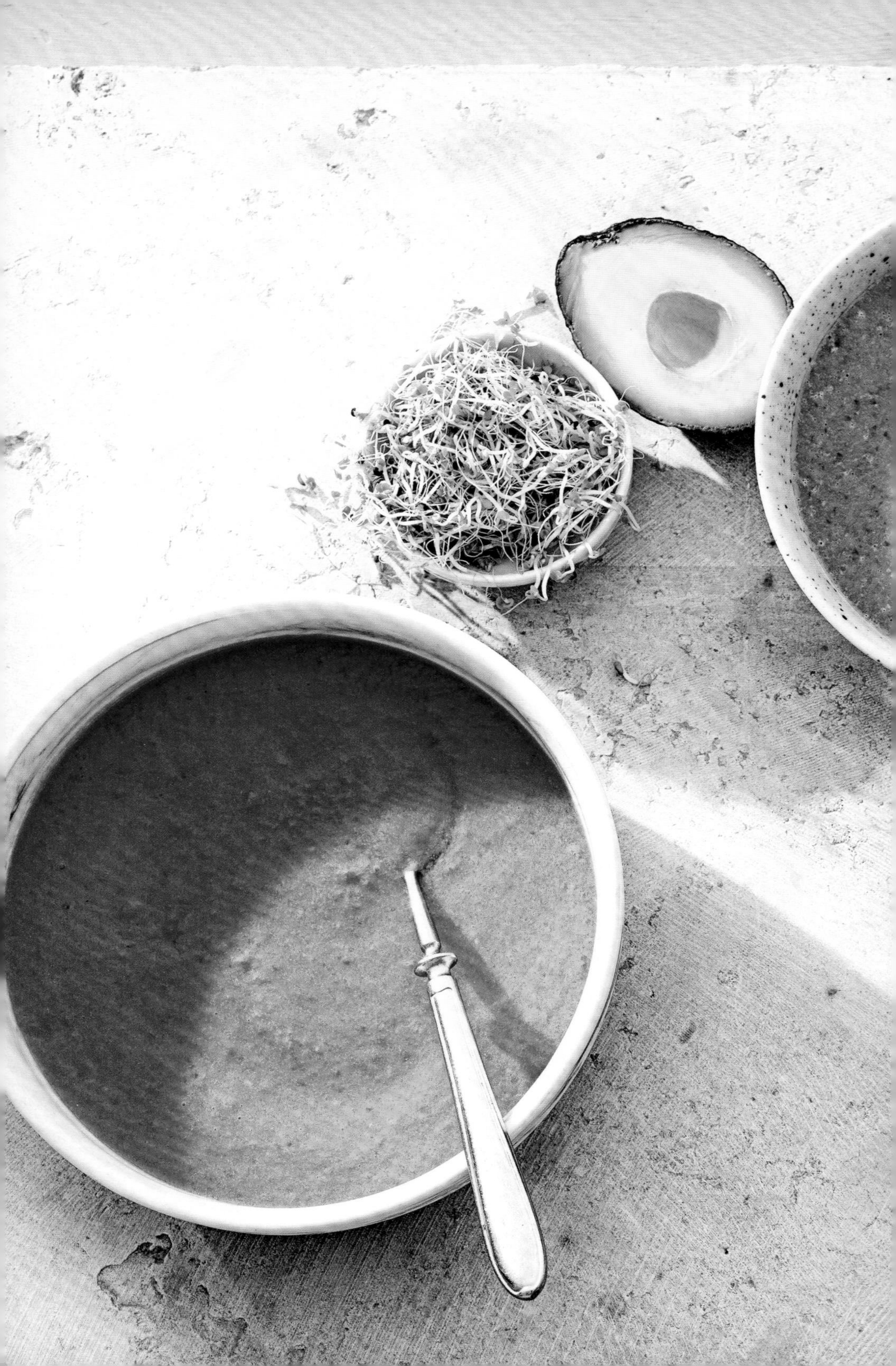

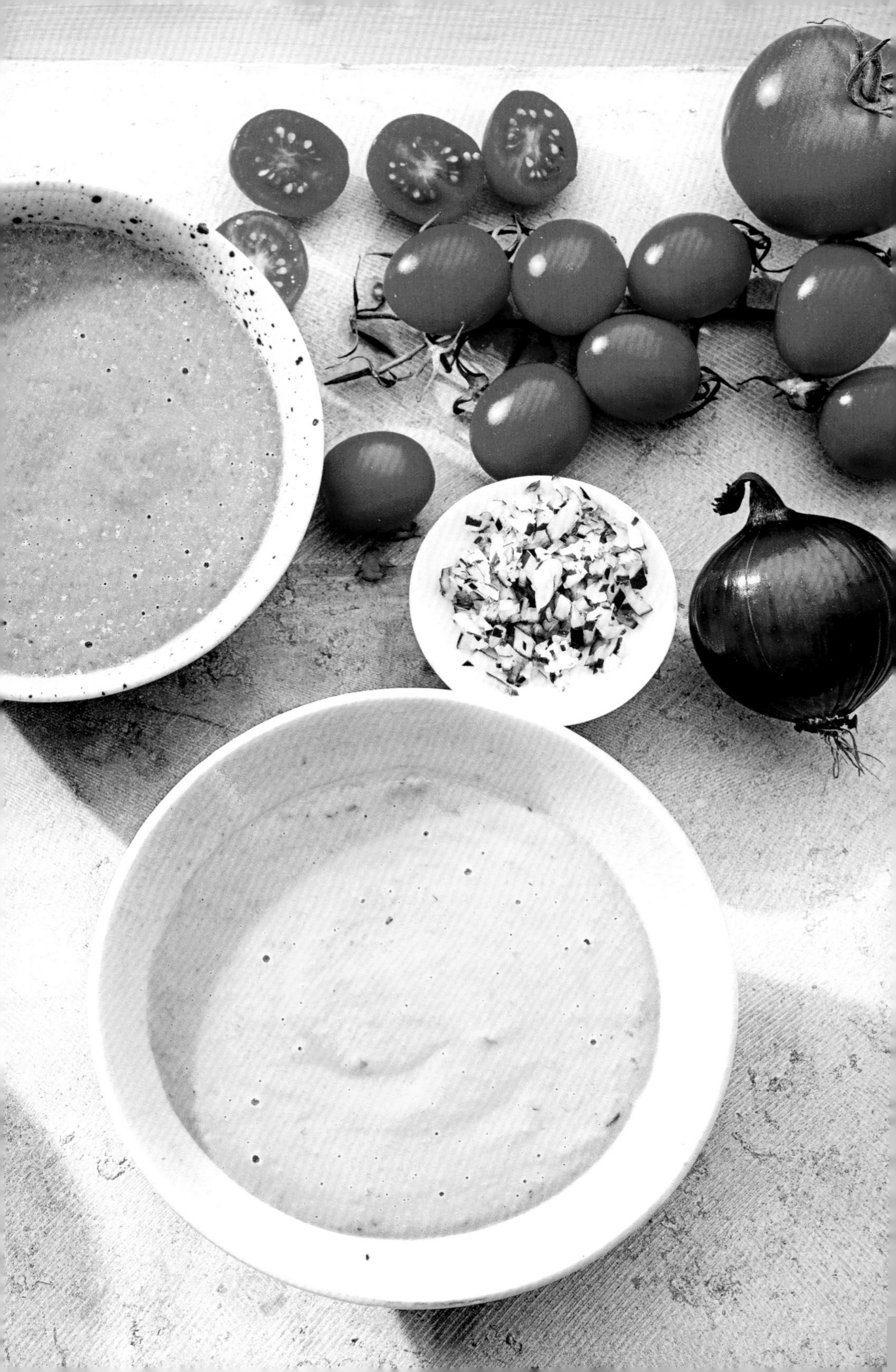

Avocado Soup

SERVES 2

2 handfuls of spinach
1 avocado
1½ cup (3 dl) water or soy/almond-based milk
2 knives' edges of chili powder
1 garlic clove
2 teaspoons lemon juice

TO ACCOMPANY

1 red onion, finely chopped
½ cup (1 dl) nondairy yogurt
1 tomato, chopped
½ cup (1 dl) alfalfa sprouts

Mix the soup ingredients. Start with the avocado and some water. Taste and season with garlic, herb salt, and lemon as you go along. This is good either warm or lukewarm. Serve with small bowls of yogurt/vegetable dip.

"A VERY VERSATILE FRUIT"

Creamy Tomato Soup

SERVES 2 TO 4

6 average-sized tomatoes
1 red bell pepper
1 avocado
Fresh or dried basil and oregano
¼ to 1 garlic clove, crushed
Lemon juice
Iodized salt or Seltin
Chili pepper

Blend all ingredients in a mixer. Heat carefully to desired temperature. Enjoy this soup as a starter or main course.

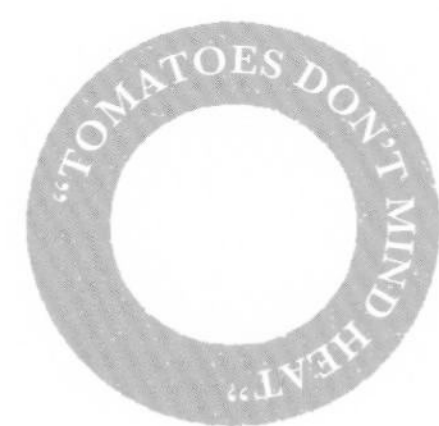

Fresh Gazpacho with Avocado

3 large avocados
2 large English cucumbers
2 large tomatoes
½–¾ cup (1–1½ dl) fresh cilantro leaves
1 medium red onion
2 large garlic cloves
1 average red chili or chili sauce of choice
½ cup (1 dl) water
3 teaspoons–1 tablespoon lime or lemon juice, freshly squeezed
1 teaspoon–1 tablespoon coconut oil or other MCT oil
1 teaspoon ionized salt
Freshly ground black pepper to taste

Cut up avocado, cucumber, tomato, and red onion into smaller pieces. Blend all ingredients in a mixer.

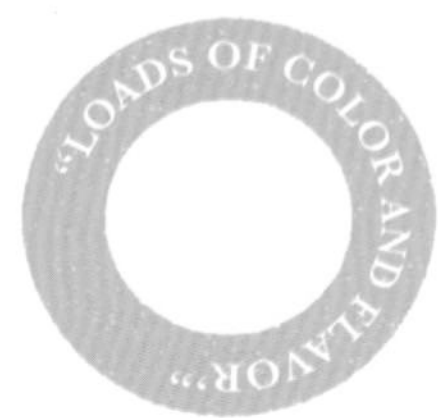

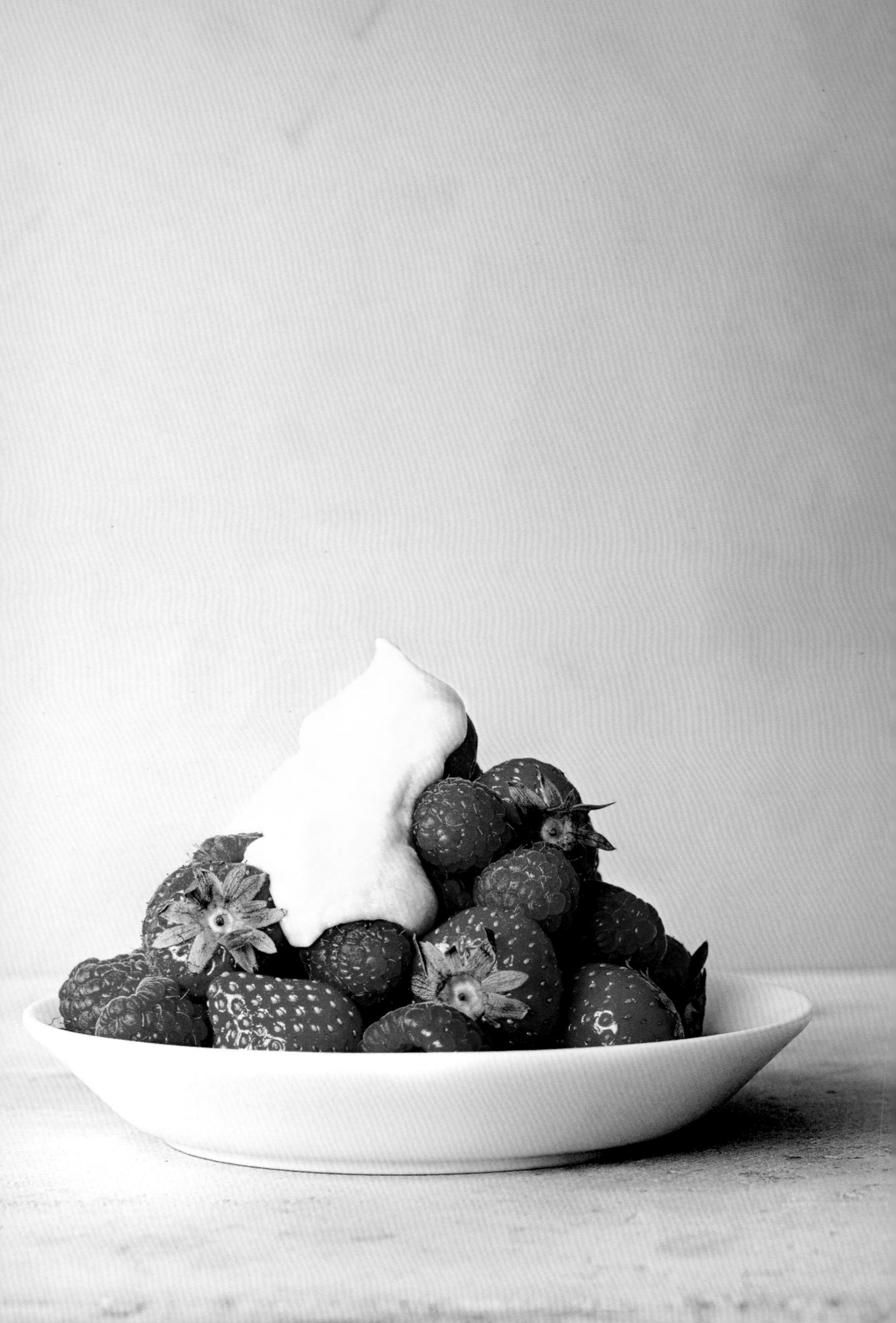

Green Cream

1 avocado
1 green banana
½ cup (1 dl) water
½ cup (1 dl) coconut oil
⅕ teaspoon (1 krm) iodized salt or Seltin

Here is a cream made of two of our favorites, avocado and green banana. Mix avocado and banana pieces, add water, and blend to a nice smooth consistency.

Add a dollop of the cream to your fruit and berries! Or season the cream to your taste with chili or herbs and use it as thickener or as an addition to savory dishes. Using mild flavoring, you can also dilute the cream into a beverage. It will keep for about three days in the refrigerator.

Alternatives to dairy cream and milk: As you have seen, it is very easy to make a healthy nondairy cream—and healthy nondairy milk!

To make cream, mix oats, cooked soybeans, almonds, or similar with water following the proportions in the above recipe. Just increase the water amount if you want milk! By all means add cashews, sesame seeds, or other nuts.

All ingredients are quickly blended to a smooth liquid in a blender. If you have a very powerful blender, the mixture is usable immediately—perhaps as cream, or if thinner, as milk in food preparation. You might have to strain the liquid if your blender is less powerful.

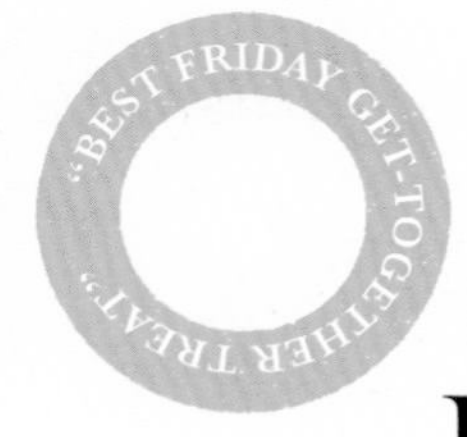

Simple Sticky Cake Loaded with Berries

PIECRUST

¾ cup (1½ dl) cashews or other nuts

¾ cup (1½ dl) coconut flakes

⅓–¾ cup (¾–1½ dl) dates

FILLING

1½ cup (3 dl) cashews

1½–3 cups (3–6 dl) strawberries or raspberries, fresh or frozen

⅓ cup (¾ dl) coconut oil or other MCT oil—try half of each

Agave syrup

⅛ cup (¼ dl) lemon or lime juice, freshly squeezed

Ground Ceylon cinnamon

Ground nutmeg

Iodized salt or Seltin

Mix the nuts and coconut flakes into a doughlike mixture. Add the dates and mix for another 3 minutes. Cover the bottom and sides of a pie pan with the dough.

Place all the filling ingredients, except the berries, in a mixer or food processor. Mix until you have a soft mixture. Add the whole or mashed berries.

Fill the the piecrust with the filling and serve immediately, or refrigerate for a later occasion.

Raw Food Chocolate Mousse

1 large avocado

1 banana, as unripe as possible

3 tablespoons coconut oil or other MCT oil

4 tablespoons cacao powder

2 tablespoons honey (no more)

Iodized salt or Seltin

Mix everything thoroughly in a blender and pour the mousse into individual bowls. Refrigerate for at least one hour before serving.

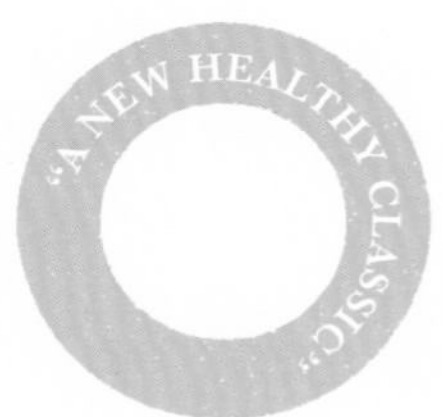

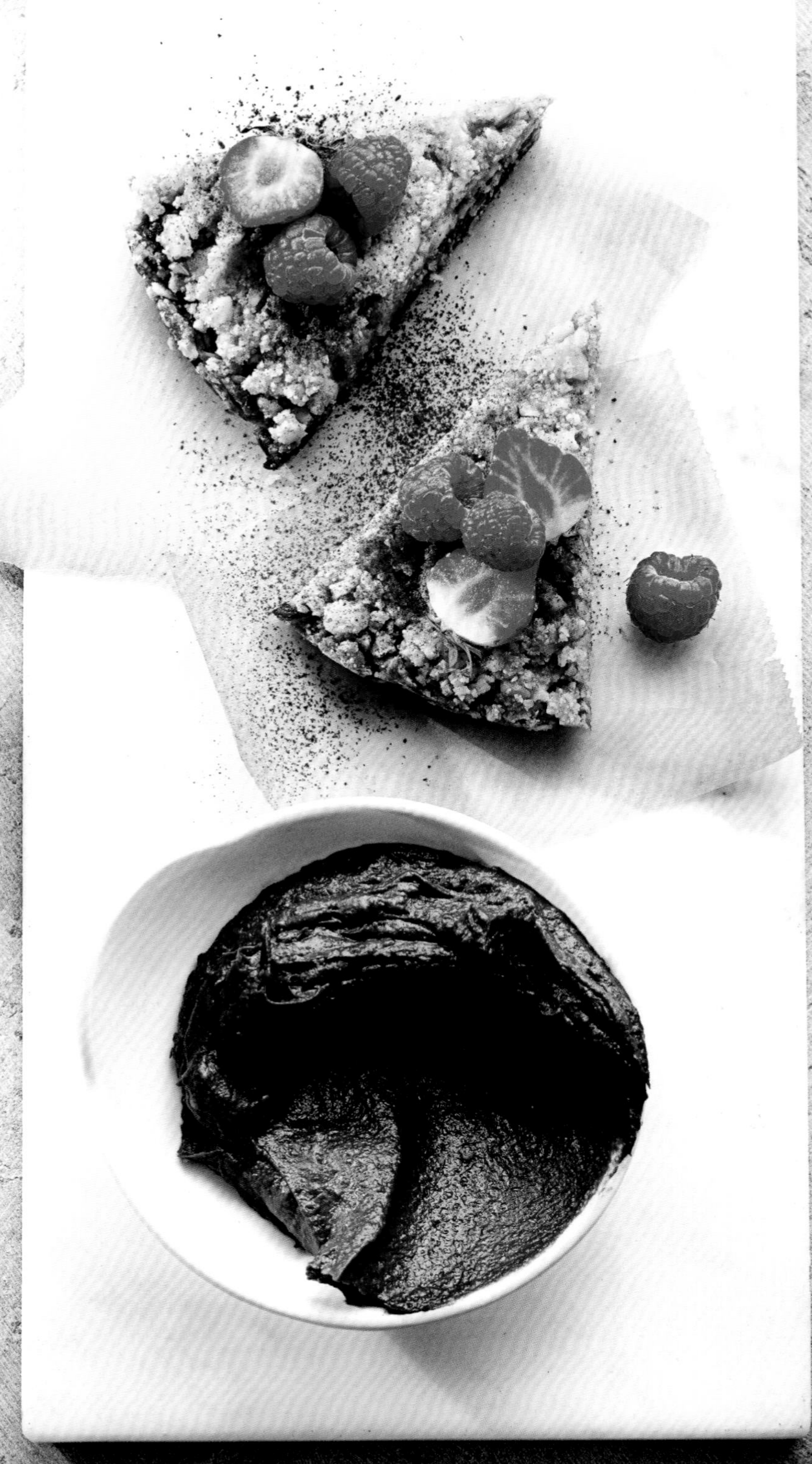

From Our Healthy Kitchen to Yours—a Collection of Tips

Let me pass on to you some of our very efficient basic tips to make your healthy eating fun and not too difficult to achieve. They sometimes overlap my twelve commandments, but that might work as a good reminder!

- Avoid industrially produced and processed foods at all costs—especially fractioned, calorie-condensed products rich in sugar and fat.
- Carefully check for additives in the foodstuff you're looking to buy. Avoid produce containing dehydrated ingredients and foods based on gene manipulation (GMO).
- The base for this dietary way of eating is all kinds of raw vegetables. They should preferably be fresh, or perhaps flash-frozen and thawed. Broccoli, arugula, spinach, and kale are all rich in antioxidants. Don't forget to add fermented vegetables like sauerkraut to your meals—they are rich in good bacteria, vitamins, antioxidants, and fiber. You can eat beans, peas, and lentils daily. Root vegetables are excellent food.
- Nearly all vegetables are most beneficial when consumed raw. If you still want to cook your beans or oven-bake root vegetables or potatoes, make sure they are lightly prepared (just a minute or two) or quickly fried. Heat carefully: low-temperature baking in the oven; quick, light stir-fry; short steaming and never use a microwave oven except to heat water.
- Above all, let the vegetables cool down before you eat them—this lowers the sugar content and promotes fiber content.
- Herbs and spices should be eaten fresh or as dried leaves. Be generous with seasonings! Instead of just decorating a dish with

a sprinkle of parsley, load the salad with parsley. Limit salt to 1 teaspoon for a plateful of food. Make sure the salt is iodized.

- Supplement your vegetarian diet with a generous amount of nuts and almonds.
- Make it fun to chop, slice, shred, and grate the vegetables! A powerful food processor is a boon in a healthy kitchen. It can make all the difference for children if you serve a festive meal where the raw beet and zucchini (with the help of a spiralizer) are presented as fluffy spaghetti strand clouds. Fennel, carrot, and radish are more delicious sliced superthin.
- Avoid cooking oils like canola and olive oil, too, even though it says "extra virgin." Instead use medium-chain fatty acids like coconut oil or MCT oil.
- Reduce or even avoid dairy products altogether, especially foods containing powdered milk. Instead use "milks" that don't come from the dairy farm: oat milk, and oat cream, soy milk, soy cheese (tofu), soy ice cream, rice milk, and similar products.
- Go easy on meat and never eat it fried or grilled. Prepare it in the oven on low temperature or cook it in red wine. We ought to avoid all fatty meat (pork as well as some cuts of beef), and concentrate on fowl, predominantly turkey. I suggest you stay away from all meat presented as sausage, meatballs, and hamburgers.
- However, you can eat fresh fish to your heart's content, especially wild-caught sea and clean freshwater fish. Prepare fish as carefully as meat. Eat the fish raw or prepare it as tartar; or marinate in lemon and serve as ceviche. Avoid farmed fish.
- If you want to consume grains, avoid the commonly available ones as their nutritional value has dramatically declined through so-called plant breeding. Use oats, buckwheat, perhaps original wheat. Why not use spelt flour, also known as dinkel? Optimal is to use grains like the African durrah or South American quinoa.
- Prioritize omega-3 and vitamin D if you want to use supplements.

Glossary

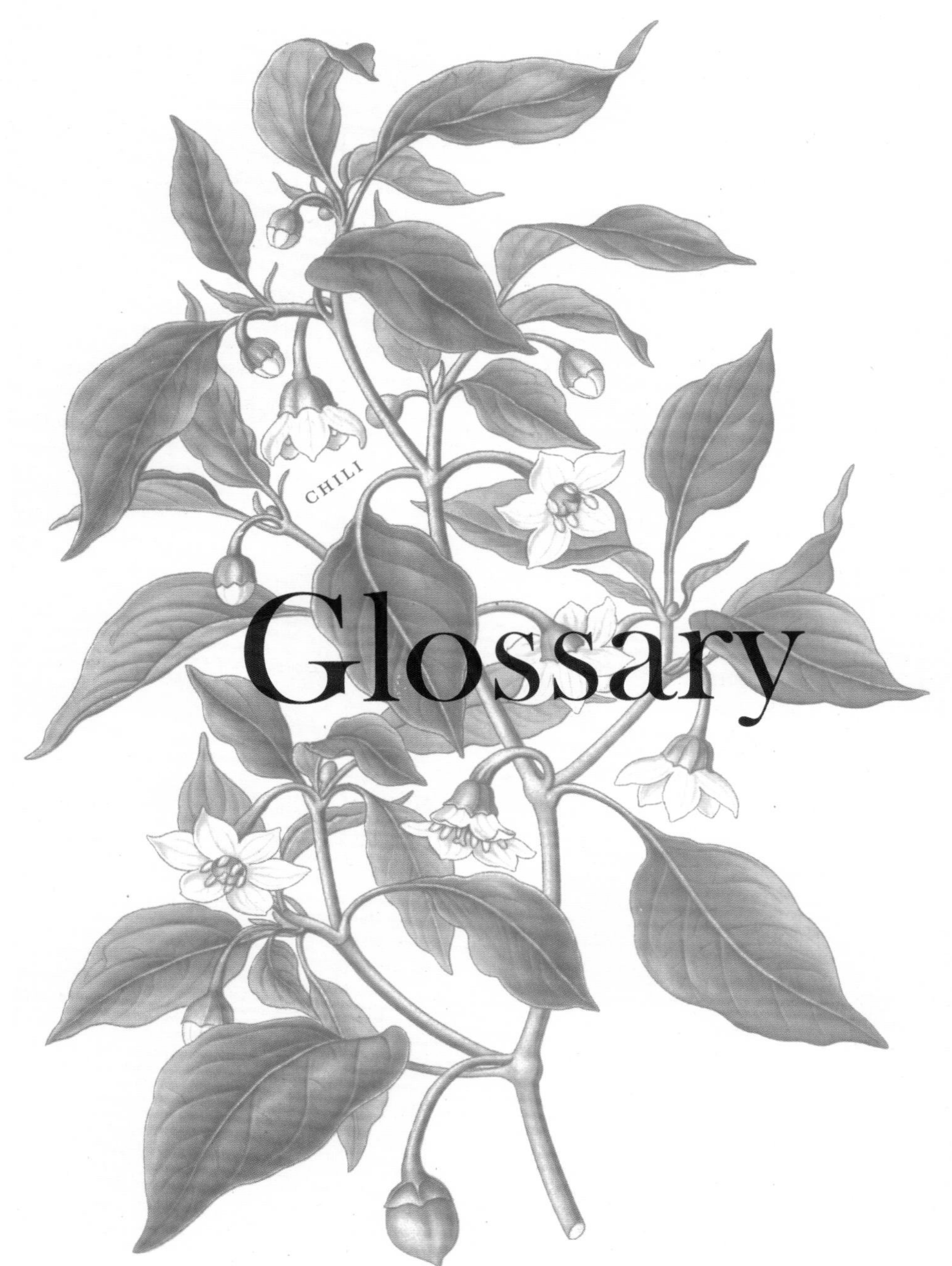

Acute phase response (APR): Acute phase reaction; early physiological defense to injury, infection, stress, tumor growth and inflammation.

ADT (androgen deprivation therapy): Abbreviation usually used in hormone treatment for prostate cancer. In our text, however, the letters stand for the "miracle grains" amaranth, durrah, and teff.

Allergens: Substances provoking allergic reactions.

Amaranth: A grain that is naturally rich in vitamins, minerals, fiber, and high-quality protein. Amaranth is used in baking and cooking, and its origin is South America.

Anti-inflammatory: Counteracts or calms inflammation.

Bacteroidetes: A phylum of Gram-negative bacteria in the gut that can prevent the development of obesity. *Firmicutes* and *Bacteroidetes* are the major phyla of bacteria in the human microbiota.

Calorie restriction (CR): Reducing calorie intake below habitual intake.

Cardiovascular disease: A collective name for diseases involving heart and blood vessels, for example, myocardial infarction (heart attack), heart failure, angina and cerebral hemorrhage (stroke), that is, blood clot or bleeding in the brain.

Chronic inflammation: Inflammation is the body's defense against infections, injury, and foreign bodies. Chronic inflammation, also called quiet or low-grade inflammation, is a condition that is believed to be the precursor for many of our common lifestyle illnesses and also many chronic illnesses.

Chronic phase response (CPR): The acute phase response turns chronic. The condition deteriorates resulting from a lack of treatment and this causes chronic illness.

COX-2: This is an enzyme involved in many cellular processes, for example, prostaglandin synthesis, a cause of inflammation.

Deadly quartet, the: Collective term for obesity, elevated cholesterol, hypertension, and glucose intolerance.

Durrah (*Sorghum bicolor*): This is a plant from the grass family. Traditionally durrah has a wide range of uses. It is used for food and animal feed, as well as to ferment alcoholic beverages. It is very useful for gluten-free baking. Durrah is the fifth most cultivated grain in the world.

Dysbiosis: This is an imbalance between good and bad—illness-causing—gut bacteria.

Early-onset coronary artery disease: Traditionally heart attacks and other acute heart problems were mostly seen in the older population, but current global studies show that it is now affecting many younger adults. Early-onset coronary artery disease is defined as fifty-five years or younger. Smoking and being overweight are among the contributing factors.

Early-onset diabetes: Type 2 diabetes usually affects the older population, but the incidence of this diagnosis in the age-group thirty to forty years old has increased globally.

Ecobiologicals: Anti-inflammatory vegetation/plants

Endotoxin: A toxic substance present in Gram-negative bacteria that is released when the bacteria dies.

ESRD (end-stage renal disease): Far-advanced kidney disease that demands dialysis or kidney transplant.

The Fat Switch: The book *The Fat Switch* by Richard J. Johnson was published by Mercola Publishing in 2012. The book discusses the reason for being overweight, how obesity can be prevented, and how through a change in diet and lifestyle you can avoid gaining weight.

Fecal microbial transplantion (FMT): A method whereby healthy bacteria from a donor's intestinal microbiota is transferred to restore an unhealthy person's microbiota. By collecting and transferring healthy bacteria from donated feces, the microbiota balance can be restored in the recipient.

Female athlete triad: A condition suffered by many female athletes. Wrong nutrition in combination with intensive physical activity can provoke hormonal disturbances with menstrual dysfunction and decreased bone density as a result.

Fermented: Raw ingredients are broken down in a metabolic process. Healthy bacteria are created and produce lactic acid and carbonic acid. Consumption of fermented foods improves the gut microbiome and the bioavailability of nutrients.

Fibromyalgia: This is a disorder characterized by chronic and generalized pain and tenderness, sleep disturbance, and fatigue. The pain is predominantly felt in the muscles, but joint pain can also be present.

Firmicutes: A phylum of bacteria where the majority have Gram-positive cell wall structure and can promote obesity. *Firmicutes* and *Bacteroidetes* are the major phyla of bacteria in the human microbiota.

GMO (genetically modified organisms): Organisms that have been modified genetically to produce desired properties.

Hemodialysis (blood dialysis): A treatment when the kidneys have completely or partially stopped working. The blood is extracted and cleaned through a filter in a dialysis machine. Wastes are removed, and the cleaned blood is returned to the body again.

IBS (irritable bowel syndrome): A disorder of the stomach-intestinal system where the intestine's motility pattern is disturbed. IBS causes stomach pain, constipation, diarrhea and often bloating and flatulence.

Lactobacillus paracasei: This is a species of Lactobacillus that is found in the gut microbiome in healthy individuals and also in fermented foodstuff. It is used in probiotics (see Probiotics).

Lactobacillus plantarum: A species of rod-shaped lactic acid bacteria that are used in probiotics (see Probiotics).

Lymphatic organs: Lymph nodes, spleen, thymus, and other lymphatic tissue, for example, tonsils and adenoids. One of the functions of the lymphatic system is to protect the body against infections.

Neurodegenerative diseases: An umbrella term for conditions that primarily affect the brain's neurons. Neurons are the nervous system's building blocks and are found in the brain and in the spinal cord. Neurons do not normally reproduce or replace themselves. If they are injured or killed, the body cannot replace them. Parkinson's disease, Alzheimer's disease, ALS (amyotrophic lateral sclerosis), and Huntington's chorea are examples of neurodegenerative diseases.

Oligosaccharides: A form of medium-long carbohydrates that function as dietary fiber and are important for feeding our colon bacteria.

Omega-3: This polyunsaturated essential fatty acid is necessary for good health and has anti-inflammatory properties. Krill, a tiny shrimp, is an important source of omega-3. This fatty acid can also be found in fatty fish like salmon, mackerel, sill and sardines, some algae, walnuts, etc.

Omega-6: This is a type of polyunsaturated fatty acid found in corn oil, sunflower oil, soy oil, sesame seed and oil, and canola oil.

Oxidative stress: A chemical imbalance created inside the body when the body produces too much harmful oxygen primarily as free radicals or when the body takes in harmful substances, like what is found in, for example, cigarette smoke.

Parabens: A family of chemicals commonly used as preservatives in hygiene products, cosmetics, and cleaning products. Artificial preservatives are used in many water-containing products to prevent bacteria and mold from forming.

Peritoneal dialysis (bag dialysis): This is a treatment when the kidneys have completely or to a major part stopped functioning. In this method the patient's own peritoneum is used as a dialysis filter. The abdominal cavity is filled with dialysis fluid through a surgically inserted catheter. The fluid is changed several times a day.

Pesticide: A toxic substance used to kill insects.

Phthalates: Chemical structures (i.e., salts or esters of phthalic acid). This is used as a plasticizer in polymers (plaster of paris) and PVC (polyvinyl chloride).

Postprandial inflammation: A destructive process created by too much fat and sugar in the blood and a strong increase of inflammation-causing toxins in the body, for example, the bacterial toxin endotoxin in the colon. An important increase in inflammation-provoking neurotransmitters is also present in the bloodstream as well as an accumulation of white blood cells—the more sugar, the stronger the reaction.

Prebiotics: These are complex carbohydrates in fiber form that are not digested by the digestive enzymes so they reach the colon intact. Prebiotics work to feed the probiotic bacteria and stimulate their proliferation.

Probiotics: These are the "good bacteria" that improve the microbiome. They often belong to the active group of lactic acid bacteria, for example, lactobacillus and bifidobacterium. The WHO defines probiotics as follows: "live organisms which when administered in adequate amounts confer a health benefit on the host."

Proinflammatory cytokines: These are proteins/signaling molecules produced by the immune system and released when there is injury, stress, or inflammation.

Scleroderma, also systemic sclerosis: This affects women more than men. The immune system mistakenly attacks the body's own cells, causing the body to produce excessive connective tissue that can accumulate in the skin, internal organs, and blood vessels. The most common sign is thickened and stiff, tight skin.

Synbiotics: A mixture of good bacteria (probiotics) and dietary fibers (prebiotics).

Teff (*Eragrostis tef*): This grain originates in Eritrea and Ethiopia. It is rich in protein, fiber, and important minerals. It is useful for making porridge or baking.

Uremic toxins: These are usually filtered and secreted by healthy kidneys. They accumulate in CKD (chronic kidney disease), when the kidneys no longer manage to filter and excrete toxins along with the urine.

My Most Sincere Thank-You

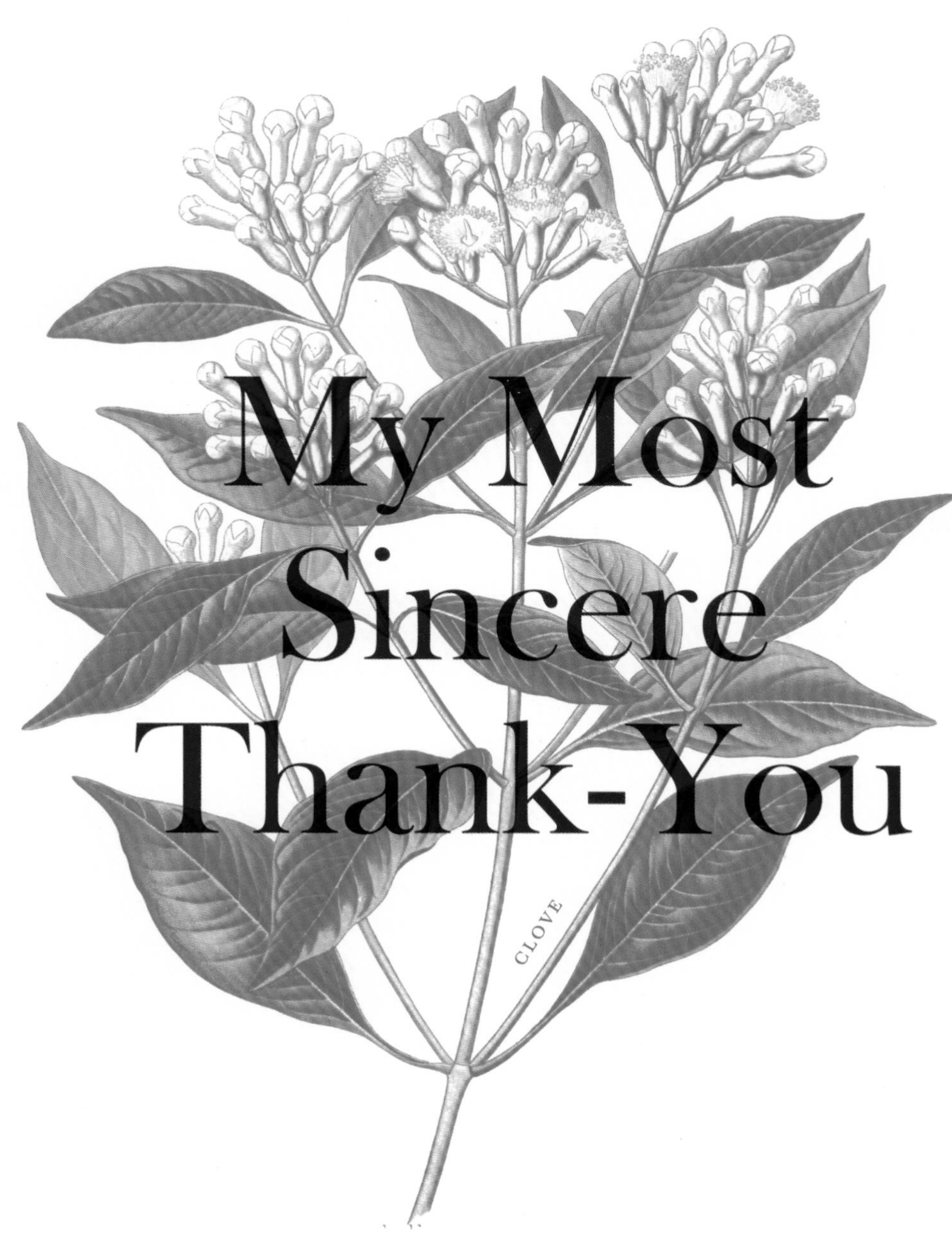

I WANT TO THANK life for all it has given me! I was born into a family where, two hundred years earlier, the children couldn't all go out together in the winter because there weren't enough shoes or slippers to go around.

As I started to say, I saw daylight on a wonderful day in April 1929; I was the firstborn in a family who lived in a small apartment above the small Pentecostal chapel in Östervåla, about thirty-one miles north of Uppsala, Sweden.

My paternal grandfather left the poverty of Matteröd in the Göinge community, which is in north Skåne, the southern part of Sweden. He became a tramcar driver in Helsingborg. He was all about moderation and modesty from early on. As a conscript, he is supposed to have earned twenty-one Swedish crowns while doing this obligatory military service, and out of that sum he saved nineteen crowns.

When I was a small child, I wanted to go with my grandfather in his tramcar between Senderö and Råå—not just once, but back and forth many times. Every time he turned the tramcar around he brought out his purse and placed a token in the payment box. He couldn't imagine that the employer should let his grandchild travel for free.

My maternal grandparents were also poor crofters—in Misterhult, between the towns of Västervik and Oskarshamn. However, this place seemed to be so far away from where we lived that I never got to meet them.

Before my father Harry, born in 1899, got the calling to teach the gospel, he trained as a landscape gardener on the Danish peninsula Jutland. At that time such a school didn't exist in Sweden and probably nowhere else in the Nordic countries. Landscape architect would be the equivalent today.

Throughout his life my father had a keen interest in plants and their important health-giving properties. This inspired me early on to take an interest in a healthy lifestyle with wholesome foods. My mother, born Berta Carlsson, also did everything to start me off right, feeding me mashed fresh vegetables long before I could chew. Nearly ninety years later, I'm certain that my health still profits from her contribution. I honor my parents' memory and all the ones gone before me. I do this every day.

My parents chose poverty, which did not offer many possibilities for further studies for my siblings and me. We were told early on that our parents would do their best to pay for our schooling through junior high. My brother, two years younger, decided to enlist; and I wanted to become a teacher. When I was sixteen years old, I applied to the teaching training college in Gothenburg but was not admitted.

Without the reforms instituted by Sweden's legendary socialist prime ministers Per-Albin Hansson and later Tage Erlander, I would never have had the opportunity to finish high school. Among the reforms was abolition of tuition fees. Combined with scholarships, like money for food and lodging and a smaller donation of three thousand Swedish Crowns through the testament of a landowner in the town of Oxelösund, I finished my education and was set on my road. I've made Tage Erlander's motto "Towards New Bold Goals" my own. I repeat it often in this time that seems to lack political vision and in a community where many seem to have lost hope.

I want to thank Bitte, my first wife and the mother of my six children. I also want to thank my children Camilla, Annette, Thomas, David, Cecilia, and Samuel for their understanding and support throughout the years. They are now ready to carry the Synbiotic part of my life's work.

I especially want to thank Marianne, my wife of nearly thirty-six years. She has stood by me through thick and thin, all over the globe—in many successes but also often in setbacks. She has shared my interests with enthusiasm; not the least, the ones dealing with a wholesome diet. She has contributed lots of healthy recipes, some of which are included in this book.

Thanks go to Professor Ragnar Romanus at Sahlgrenska Akademin, who "discovered" and recruited me as surgeon in 1959. He put up with me for eleven years, and he gave me his absolute unconditional support.

A heartfelt thank-you to all the young graduates, PhD students, physicians in training, and surgeons who choose to study and advance in my environment—not least the 120 doctoral candidates I mentored in research, examined, and frequently also tutored.

A very special thank-you goes to my close collaborators during many years: the Professors Roland Andersson, Bo Eklöf, Lars-Olov Hafström, Per-Olof Hasselgren, Bengt Jeppson, Lars Norgren, Rolf Olsson, Stig Steen, Karl Tranberg, Bruno Walther, and many more who put up with all the projects I too often suggested and who helped bring many of them to successful conclusion.

It is thanks to these colleagues that I have managed to contribute in excess of a thousand scientific papers; from my humble start in 1953 with an osteologic investigation in Gudhem of Klosterkyrkan's skulls from the Middle Ages up to the present extensive project studies of ADHD children at the Karolinska hospital in Stockholm, Sweden; treatment of liver transplant recipients in Auckland, New Zealand, and the large EU-backed multicenter research study Eat2BeNice. I also give my heartfelt thanks for all contributors to this last-mentioned study. Only one, Catharina Lavebratt, mentioned by name, but absolutely no one forgotten. Catharina Lavebratt was the central figure in this research endeavor. Last but not least, I want to thank, among all my research contacts, Professor Roger Williams, head of liver research at London University. For eighteen years he provided me with a stimulating environment to work in.

Mia Clase and Lina Nertby Aurell, authors of *Food Pharmacy*, have played an indescribably important part these last few years. Today, their book has been translated into about thirty languages, and their blog with the same name has thousands of readers. The result of meeting Mia and Lina is that the knowledge I have probed for nearly seventy years, and to a certain extent based my research on, now can be shared globally.

It's with great gratitude that I present my first book written purely for the general public. It would not have been possible without the access to two top-rated "A"s—Anna Andersson, health expert, and Astrid Hasselrot, editor. Together they formed a true Triple A team that contributed enormously.

Another heartfelt thank-you goes to Volante publishing company, the perfect choice, and to the head of publishing, Tobias Nielsen; and especially to publishing editor Ulrika Bergwall, who devoted her superb skills and time to just my book. Other experts involved in the production of this book are, particularly, source editor and translator Ulla-Stina Rask. I also want to warmly thank the book's designer, Sebastian Wadsted, and Volante's Albin Grahn. Zlatan doesn't win the soccer match on his own—he needs his full team to succeed—and a full team is something Volante has really made sure that I had alongside me.

To the extent that my life's work has been a success, it mostly comes down to hard work from morning until late night. This did, unfortunately, bring about a certain lack of consideration for others' work and life constraints. This is something I sometimes have difficulty taming. To the people this has hurt, and I'm sure that there are quite a few, I hereby ask for forgiveness.

Let us all thank life! Welcome all to share my praise.

Stig Bengmark

Sources

BLACKBERRY

P. 21 *A scientific investigation by the Norwegian professor of immunology Per Brandzaeg:* Brandzaeg, P. et al., "Immunobiology and immunopathology of human gut mucosa: humoral immunity and intraepithelial lymphocytes," *Gastroenterology* 97, no. 6 (Dec. 1989): 1562–1584.

P. 24 *For liver transplant the number is more like every second patient*: "Post-OLT infections are estimated to occur in more than 50% of OLT recipients. Bacterial infections account for most post-transplant infections (up to 70%) followed by viral and fungal infections." Hernandez, M. Del Pilar, et al., "Infectious Complications After Liver Transplantation," *Gastroenterol Hepatol (NY)* 11, no. 11 (Nov. 2015): 742–753. Already in 2011, the following was found and reported in this study: "It is estimated that up to 80% of liver recipients will develop at least one infection during the first year after transplantation, and, while most are successfully treated, some will result in death. . . . Indeed, opportunistic infections are a leading cause of death during the first three years after liver transplantation," *World Journal of Hepatology* 3, no. 4 (Apr. 2011): 83–92. ncbi.nlm.nih.gov/pmc/articles/PMC3098392/.

P. 25 *Prognosis shows that "affluenza diseases"*: Between 2006 and 2016 the share of individuals in Sweden with obesity had increased by 2.8 percent in women and with 4.3 percent in men. Folkhälsomyndigheten (Public Health Authority), "Overweight and Obesity," 2016, folkhalsomyndigheter.se/folkhalsorapportering- statistik/folkhalsansutveckling/levnadsvanor/overvikt-och-fetma/. WHPA (World Health Professionals Association) warn already in 2011 of "an epidemic of chronic diseases." The so-called "nontransmissible diseases" (many are lifestyle related) increased as cause of mortality between 2008 to 2012 from 60 percent to 68 percent. Also: "These diseases have become a serious threat to humanity's health, and if action is not taken quickly this burden on the global health will continue to increase dramatically." World Health Professionals Association, "Health Professionals unite to issue warning on global epidemic of non-communicable diseases" March 16, 2011, whpa.org/WHPA_NCD_campaign_media_release_16052011.pdf.
The Lancet published a global study in April 2018 that showed that global healthcare costs risk doubling up to year 2040. Dieleman, J. L. et al., "Trends in future health financing and coverage: future health spending and universal health coverage in 188 countries, 2016–2040," *The Lancet* 391, no. 10132 (May 2018): 1783–1798. thelancet.com/journals/lancet/article/PIIS0140-6736(18)30697-4/fulltext.

P. 26. *In conclusion, diabetes will have doubled:* Hebert, L. E. et al., "Alzheimer Disease in the US Population Prevalence Estimates Using the 2000 Census," *Archives of Neurology* 60, no. 8 (Aug. 2003): 1119–1122. In 2015, it was estimated that more than 9.9 million new cases of dementia would be diagnosed in the future, which means one new case every third second. This estimate is nearly 30 percent higher than the one made for 2010. Wimo, A. et al., "The worldwide cost of dementia 2015 and comparisons with 2010" in *Alzheimer's and Dementia* 13 (Jan. 2017): 1.

P. 26 *For example, they increased the intake of:* Gadda, T. and Gasparatos, A., "Tokyo Drifts from Seafood to Meat Eating" March 19, 2011. UNU (United Nations University), unu.edu/publications/articles/tokyo-drifts-from-seafood-to-meateating.html#info. Several studies have shown that the traditional Japanese diet with plenty of vegetables, soybeans, green tea, fish and the absence of processed foodstuffs and dairy products is an important health factor. However, obesity, diabetes, and cardiovascular disease are increasing in Japan. In 2005 the government recommended that the population keep to the traditional Japanese diet. Gabriel, A. S. et al., "The Role of the Japanese Traditional Diet in Healthy and Sustainable Patterns around the World," in *Nutrients* 10 (Feb. 2018): 2.

P. 27 *During the first fifty years:* A 2008 study of Japanese men showed a strong connection between consumption of dairy products and prostate cancer. Kurahashi, N. et al., "Dairy Product, Saturated Fatty Acid and Calcium Intake and Prostate Cancer in a Prospective Cohort of Japanese Men," *Cancer Epidemiology, Biomarkers & Prevention* 17 (Apr. 2008): 4. cebp.aacjournals.org/contents/17/4/930.

P. 28 *The prognosis for 2050 is that resistant bacteria:* A report initiated by the British government found that in 2050 more people will die yearly due to antibiotic resistance than from cancer. The Review on Antimicrobial Resistance, "Tackling drug-resistant infections globally; final report and recommendations," May 16, 2016, amr-review.org/sites/default/files/160518_Final%20paper_with%20cover.pdf.

P. 28 *It is dizzying how quickly they have increased:* "Simultaneously as the biggest threats to health during the 1900—cardiovascular disease, infectious disease and cancer—only increase marginally, there are at least forty chronic illnesses and conditions which have more than doubled in the last generation. Many weren't even on our radar before 1980." Lear, R, "The Root Cause in the Dramatic Rise of Chronic Disease," Brown University, app.box.

com/s/iyjuzrxtkx3gpblu4vmtowjrgsxykuzc. Autism (2094%), Alzheimer's (299%), COPD (148%), diabetes (305%), sleep apnea (430%), celiac disease (1111%), ADHD (819%), asthma (142%), depression (280%), bipolar disease in youth (10833%), osteoarthritis (4495), lupus (787%), inflammatory bowel disease (120%), chronic fatigue syndrome (11027%), fibromyalgia (7727%), multiple sclerosis (117%), and hypothyrodism (702%).

P. 29 *Consumption of 1 3/4 lbs (800 g) of fruit and vegetables:* Aune, D. et al., "Fruit and vegetable intake and the risk of cardiovascular disease, total cancer and all-cause mortality—a systematic review and dose-responsive metaanalysis of prospective studies," *International Journal of Epidemiology* 46, no. 3 (June 2017): 1029–1056.

P. 30 *The simple answer is that Stone Age people:* Robbins, J. *Healthy at 100: The Scientifically Proven Secrets of the World's Healthiest and Longest-Lived Peoples*, New York: Random House, 2006.

P. 31 *Recently reported in Great Britain:* "Failing to address the challenge posed by the obesity epidemic will place an even greater burden on NHS resources. It is estimated that the NHS spent £6.1 billion on overweight and obesity-related ill-health in 2014 to 2015. Annual spend on the treatment of obesity and diabetes is greater than the amount spent on the police, the fire service and the judicial system combined." Public Health England, "Scale of the obesity problem," March 31, 2017, gov.uk/government/publications/health-matters-obesity-and- the-food-environment—2.

P. 32 *The level of inflammation a meal:* Erridge, C. et al., "A high-fat meal induces low-grade endotoxemia: evidence of a novel mechanism of postprandial inflammation," *American Journal of Clinical Nutrition* 86, no. 5 (Oct. 2007): 1286–1292.

P. 53 *When the calorie intake for rats and mice was reduced*: Picca, A. et al., "Does eating less make you live longer and better? An update on calorie restriction," *Clinical Interventions in Aging* 12 (2017): 1887–1902.

P. 53 *Few studies have been done on humans*: Hy, S. et al., "A calorie-restriction diet supplemented with fish oil and high-protein powder is associated with reduced severity of metabolic syndrome in obese women," *European Journal of Clinical Nutrition* 69, no. 3 (Mar. 2015): 322–328.

P. 58 *The book* Physica *is all about health and healing:* Von Bingen, H., *Physica, The Complete English Translation of Her Classic Work on Health and Healing*, trans. Priscilla Throop. Rochester, VT: Inner Traditions, 1998.

P. 60 *Many new synthetic substances start to form at 176°F (80°C):* Grootveld, M. et al., "Long-chain and medium-chain fatty acids—effects of heating," *Journal of Food Service* 13, no. 1 (Oct. 2001): 41–55.

P. 60 *According to the American Lung Association*: American Lung Association, "What's in a cigarette?," lung.org/stop-smoking/smoking-facts/what-in-a-cigarette.html.

P. 61 *The French scientist Louis Camille Maillard suggested in the 1900s:* Maillard's discoveries are collected under the designation Maillard reactions, see "Maillard reactions," food-info.net/uk/colour/maillard.htm. There have recently been several follow-up studies. See Zhang, Q., et al., "A Perspective on the Maillard Reaction and the Analysis of Protein Glycation by Mass Spectrometry: Probing the Pathogenesis of Chronic Disease," *Journal of Proteome Research* 8, no. 2 (Feb. 2009): 754–769.

P. 63 *Antioxidant-rich foods:* "USDA Database for the Oxygen Radical Absorbance Capacity (ORAC) of Selected Foods," Release 2, U.S. Department of Agriculture, May 2010, orac-info-portal.de/download/ORAC_R2.pdf.

P. 68 *An animal study published in 2017*: "Supplementation with Omega-3 fatty acids can counteract imbalance in the gut biome, lower levels of endotoxins in the blood through the portal vein and improve weight." Cao, Z. J. et al., "Effect of n-3 polyunsaturated fatty acids on gut microbiota and endotoxin levels in portal vein of rats fed with a high-fat diet" in *Zongguo yi xue ke xue yuan xue bao. Axta Academiae Medicinae Sinicae* 36, no. 5 (Oct. 2014): 496–500.

P. 68 *Even though sunflower oil and olive oil are long-chain:* Yu, S. et al., "In Vitro Evidence of Anti-Inflammatory and Anti-Obesity Effects of Medium-Chain Fatty Acid-Diacylglycerols," *Journal of Microbiology and Biotechnology* 27, no. 9 (Sept. 2017): 1617–1627.

P. 68 *Krill oil also contains:* Burri, L. et al., "Differential Effects of Krill Oil and Fish Oil on the Hepatic Transcriptome in Mice," *Frontiers in Genetics* 2 (July 2011): 45.

P. 69 *Regular consumption of omega-3*: Ellulu, M. S. et al., "Role of fish oil in human health and possible mechanism to reduce the inflammation," *Inflammopharmacology* 23, no. 2–3 (Feb. 2015): 79–89.

P. 72 *Studies show that the majority*: Several studies were performed for the specific groups. The more common example is the study by Daudi, N. et al., "Evaluation of Vitamin D deficiency in hospitalized patients in Brussels," *Revue Medicale de Bruxelles* 30, no. 1 (Jan 2009): 5–10. The study found that more than 60 percent of the examined patients hospitalized for acute conditions had noticeable vitamin D deficiency.

P. 72 *An American-European research project*: Gant, W. B. et al., "Estimated benefit of increased vitamin D status in reducing the economic burden of disease in Western Europe," *Progress in Biophysics & Molecular Biology* 99, no. 2–3 (Feb.–Apr. 2009): 104–113.

P. 84 *Studies have actually shown*: Ristow, M. et al., "Antioxidants prevent health-promoting effects of physical exercise in humans," *Proc Natl Acad Sci USA* 106, no. 21 (May 2009): 8665–8670.

P. 85 . . . *describing how a phenomenon*: Mallinson, R. J. and Souza, M. J. De "Current perspectives on the etiology and manifestation of the 'silent' component of the Female Athlete Triad," *International Journal of Women's Health* 6 (May 2014): 496–500.

P. 85 *So far there has been little evidence*: Costa e Silva, L. et al., "Physical Activity-Related Injury Profile in Children and Adolescents According to Their Age, Maturation and Level of Sports Participation," *Sports Health* 9, no. 2 (Mar.–Apr. 2017): 118–125.

P. 86 *Alzheimer's disease*: Farina, N. et al., "The effect of exercise interventions on cognitive outcome in Alzheimer's disease: a systematic review," *International Psychogeriatrics* 26, no. 1 (Jan. 2014): 9–18.

P. 86 *ADHD*: Pan, C. Y. et al., "Effects of Physical Exercise Intervention on Motor Skills and Executive Functions in Children with ADHD: a Pilot Study," *Journal of Attention Disorders* (Feb. 2015).

P. 86 *Diabetes*: Melmer, A. et al., "The Role of Physical Exercise in Obesity and Diabetes," *Praxis* 107, no. 17–18 (Aug. 2018): 971–976.

P. 86 *Breast cancer*: Gonçalves, A. K. et al., "Effects of physical activity on breast cancer prevention: a systematic review," *Journal of Physical Activity and Health* 11, no. 2 (Feb. 2014): 445–454.

P. 86 *Prostate cancer*: Richman, E. L. et al., "Physical activity after diagnosis and risk of prostate cancer progression: data from the cancer of prostate strategic urologic research endeavor," *Cancer Research* 71, no. 11 (June 2011): 3889–3895.

P. 86 *The very best result:* Nguyen, J. Y., "Adoption of a plant-based diet by patients with recurrent prostate cancer," *Integrative Cancer Therapies* 5, no. 6 (Sept. 2006): 214–225.

P. 90 *A recently performed examination*: Kim, M. J., et al., "Fate and complex pathogenic effects of dioxins and polychlorinated biphenyls in obese subjects before and after drastic weight loss," *Environmental Health Perspective* 119, no. 3 (March 2011): 377–383.

P. 91 *It was observed already 50 years ago*: Jaeger, R. J., "Migration of a Phthalate Ester Plasticizer from Polyvinyl Chloride Blood Bags into Stored Human Blood and Its Localization in Human Tissues," *New England Journal of Medicine* 287, no. 22 (Nov. 1972): 1114–1118.

P. 91 *Alcohol abuse arrives first in tenth place*: Danaei, G. et al., "The preventable causes of death in the United States: comparative risk assessment of dietary, lifestyle, and metabolic risk factors," *PLos Medicine* 6 (April 2009): 4.

P. 91 *Scientists today talk about:* For more on "The Deadly Quartet," see: Bengmark, S., "Obesity, the deadly quartet and the contribution of the neglected daily organ rest—a new dimension of un-health and its prevention," from *Hepatobiliary Surgery and Nutrition* 4, no. 4 (Aug. 2015): 278–288.

P. 94 *Communication between digestive organs*: Mayer, E. A., "Gut microbes and the brain: paradigm shift in neuroscience," *Journal of Neuroscience* 34, no. 46 (Nov. 2014): 15490–15496.

P. 100 *Large investigations*: World Cancer Research Fund International, "Limit red and processed meat," 2018, wcrf.org/dietandcancer/recommendations/limit-red-processed-meat.

P. 100 *Global meat consumption*: Jordbruksverket (2018).

P. 101 *For example, India*: World Cancer Research Fund International, "Limit red and processed meat," 2018.

P. 102 *A renowned American investigation*: Fontana, L., et al., "Long-term low-calorie low-protein vegan diet and endurance exercise are associated with low cardiometabolic risk," *Rejuvenation Research* 10, no. 2 (June 2007): 225–234.

P. 104 *Research shows that calves*: Hostettler-Allen, L., et al., "Insulin resistance, hyperglycemia, and glucosuria in intensively milk-fed calves," *Journal of Animal Science* 72, no. 1 (Jan. 1994): 160–173.

P. 105 *In one study performed in North America*: Pan, A. et al., "Red Meat Consumption and Mortality: Results From 2 Prospective Cohort Studies," *Archives of Internal Medicine* 172, no. 7 (2012): 555–563.

P. 106 *In the second study*: Rohrmann, S. et al., "Meat consumption and mortality— results from the European Prospective Investigation into Cancer and Nutrition," *BMC Medicine* 11 (Mar. 2013): 63.

P. 110 World Facts, "Countries who consume the most cheese," worldatlas.com/articles/countries-who-consume-the-most- cheese.html.

P. 112 *The insemination technique has resulted in*: Arla, "Konsumentkontakt" (customer service), Response to the question "How often is a cow calving?" September 27, 2017, konsumentkontakt.arla.se/org/arla/s/hur-ofta-ar-en-ko-draktig/.

P.114 *Breast cancer mortality in a country*: Carroll, K. K., "Experimental evidence of dietary factors and hormone-dependent cancers," *Cancer Research* 11 (Nov. 1975): 3374–3383. For follow-up studies and more information, see Carroll, K. K., "Influence of Diet on Hormone-Dependent Cancers," *Xenobiotic Metabolism: Nutritional Effects* (1985): 177–186: Carroll, K. K., "Summation: Which fat/how much fat—Animals," *Preventive Medicine* 16, no. 4 (July 1987): 510–515; Ray, A., "Cancer preventive role of selected dietary factors," *Indian Journal of Cancer* 42, no. 1 (2005): 15–24; Myles, I. A., "Fast food fever: reviewing the impacts of the Western diet on immunity," *Nutrition Journal*, June 2014.

P. 115 *An Icelandic study*: Torfadottir, J. E. et al., "Milk Intake in Early Life and Risk of Advanded Prostate Cancer," *American Journal of Epidemiology* 175, no. 2 (Jan. 2012): 144–153.

P. 115 *A robust Swedish investigation several years later*: Michaëlsson, K. et al., "Milk intake and risk of mortality and fractures in women and men: cohort studies," *British Medical Journal* (2014). Also: Spross, Å., "New Uppsala study: Excess milk may shorten life span," *Uppsala Nya Tidning* February 14, 2017, unt.se/nyheter/uppsala/nyuppsalastudie-mycket-mjolk-kan-korta-livet-4544028.aspx.

P. 118 *Scientific studies report*: See, among others, Ruuskanen, A. et al., "Postive serum antigliadin antibodies without celiac disease in the elderly population: Does it matter?," *Scandinavian Journal of Gastroenterology* 45, no. 10 (Oct. 2010): 1197–1202.

P. 118 *Consumption of gluten is associated with*: Sapone, A. et al., "Divergence of gut permeability and mucosal immune gene expression in two gluten-associated conditions: celiac disease and gluten sensitivity," *BMC Medicine* 9 (Mar. 2011).

P. 126 *Turmeric also improves regeneration*: Aggarwal, B. B., and S. Prasad, "Turmeric, the Golden Spice" from *Herbal Medicine: Biomolecular and Clinical Aspects*. CRC Press/Taylor & Francis, 2011.

P. 126 *Its anti-infective effects:* Turmeric's effect on different diseases has been the subject of many recent studies. Turmeric has, among other things, shown to ease the effect of influenza. Han, S. et al., "Curcumin ameliorates severe influenza pneumonia via attenuating lung injury and regulating macrophage cytokines productions," *Clinical and experimental pharmacology and physiology* 45, no. 1 (Jan. 2018): 84–93. The conclusion is that turmeric (curcumin) has the potential to become a promising part in the cure for Ebola. See: Baikerikar, S., "Curcumin and Natural Derivatives Inhibit Ebola Viral Proteins: An In Silico Approach," *Pharmacognosy Research* 9, no. 5 (Dec. 2017): 15–22.

P. 128 *It is a definite advantage*: Benefits of MCT fats, see Geng, S., et al., "Medium-chain triglyceride ameliorates insulin resistance and inflammation in high fat diet-induced obese mice," *European Journal of Nutrition* 55 (Apr. 2016): 931– 940; Nafar, F., et al., "Coconut oil protects cortical neurons from amyloid beta toxicity by enhancing signaling of cell survival pathways," *Neurochem International* 105 (May 2017): 64–79; Otsuka, H., et al., "Effectiveness of Medium-Chain Triglyceride Oil Therapy in Two Japanese Citrin-Deficient Siblings: Evaluation Using Oral Glucose Tolerance Test," *Tohoku Journal of Experimental Medicine* 240, no. 4 (Dec. 2016): 323–328.

P. 129 *Clinical studies have shown that the intake of at least one avocado a day*: Fulgoni, V. L, et al., "Avocado consumption is associated with better diet quality and nutrient intake, and lower metabolic syndrome risk in US adults: results from the National Health and Nutrition Examination Survey (NHANES) 2001-2008," *Nutrition Journal* 12, no. 1 (Jan. 2013). nutritionj.biomedcentral.com/articles/10.1186/1475-2891-12-1.

P. 130 *The strongest effects was observed*: Vahedi, L. L., "Evaluating the effect of four extracts of avocado fruit on esophageal squamous carcinoma and colon adenocarcinoma cell lines in comparison with peripheral blood mononuclear cells," *Acta Medica Iranica* 52, no. 3 (2014): 201–205.

P. 130 *Animal tests have shown*: Boileau, C., et al., "Protective effects of total fraction of avocado/soybean unsaponifiables on the structural changes in experimental dog arthritis: inhibition of nitric oxide synthase and matrix metalloproteinase-13," *Arthritis Research & Therapy* 11, no. 2 (Mar. 2009).

P. 132 *Foods with high antioxidant content*: U.S. Department of Agriculture, "USDA Database for the Oxygen Radical Absorbance Capacity (ORAC) of Selected Foods," Release, May 2, 2010, orac-info-portal-de/download/ORAC_R2.pdf.

P. 135 *Cinnamon together with other spices*: McCrea, C. E., "Effects of culinary spices and psychological stress on postprandial lipemia and lipase activity: results of a randomized crossover study and in vitro experiments," *Journal of Translational Medicine* 13, no. 7 (Jan. 2015).

P. 135 *Another study consisting of 22 subjects*: Ziegenfuss, T. N., et al., "Effects of a water-soluble cinnamon extract on body composition and features of the metabolic syndrome in pre-diabetic men and women," *Journal of The International Society of Sports Nutrition* 3, no. 2 (Dec. 2006): 45–53.

P. 135 *In fact, PubMed has 1500 studies*: Ranasinghe, P., et al., "Medicinal properties of 'true' cinnamon (*Cinnamomum zeylanicum*): a systematic review," *BMC Complementary and Alternative Medicine* 13 (Oct. 2013): 275.

P. 136 *Apart from all this, the chili pepper is attributed*: Anand, K. S., and V. Dhikav, "Migraine relieved by chilis," *Headache: The Journal of Head and Face Pain* 52, no. 6 (June 2012). Also: Arwa, K. K., "Topical Analgesic Nano-lipid Vesicle Formulation of Capsaicinoids Extracts of Bhut Jolokia (Capsicum chinense Jacq): Pharmacodynamic Evaluation in Rat Models and Acceptability Studies in Human Volunteers," *Current Drug Delivery* 13, no. 88 (2016): 1325–1338.

P. 139 *Cacao is most known for*: Buitrago-Lopez, A., et al., "Chocolate consumption and cardiometabolic disorders: systematic review and meta-analysis," *British Medical Journal* 343 (Aug. 2011): 4488.

P. 140, 141 *Approximately 275 articles, research reports and overviews*: Gambero, A., and M. L. Ribero, "The Positive Effect of Yerba Mate (*Ilex paraguariensis*) in Obesity," from *Nutrients* 7, no. 2 (Feb. 2015): 730–750.

P. 142 *A group of English researchers decided*: Corder, R., et al., "Oenology: red wine procyanidins and vascular health," *National Center for Biotechnology Information* 444, no. 7119 (Nov. 2006): 566.

P. 146 *These have shown to contain*: "Updated list: The world's most pesticide contaminated crops," Aktuell Hållbarhet, April 19, 2018, aktuellhallbarhet.se/ny-lista--varldens-mest-besprutade-grodor/.

P. 147 *Dirty Dozen*: The Environmental Working Group (EWG), "Dirty Dozen," 2018, ewg.org/foodnews/dirty-dozen.php.

P. 165 *Chart*: Hatori, M., et al., "Time-restricted feeding without reducing calorie intake prevents metabolic diseases in mice fed a high-fat diet," *Cell Metabolism* 15, no. 6 (June 2012): 848–860.

P. 166 *Chart:* Chaix, A. et al., "Time-restricted feeding is a preventative and therapeutic intervention against diverse nutritional challenges," *Cell Metabolism* 20, no. 9 (Dec. 2014): 991–1005.

P. 168 *The following illnesses*: Many studies over the years show the connection between excess body weight and disease. See: Ard, J. D., "Health Risks of Overweight & Obesity," from National Institute of Diabetes and Digestive and Kidney Diseases, February 2018, niddk.hih.gov/health-information/weight-management/adult-over-weight-obesity/health-risks.

P. 169 *The fat switch*: Johnsson, R. J., *The Fat Switch*, Mercola.com: 2012

P. 170 *CR accomplishes the same health effects*: See Martin, C. K., et al., "Effect of Calorie Restriction on Mood, Quality of Life, Sleep and Sexual Function in Healthy Non-Obese Adults: The CALERIE 2 Randomized Clinical Trial," from *National Center for Biotechnology Information* 176, no. 6 (June 2016): 743–752; Golbidi, S., "Health Benefits of Fasting and Caloric Restrictions," *Current Diabetes Report* 17, no. 12 (Oct. 2017): 123.

P. 177 *He was the first person who*: Burkitt, D. P., *Don't Forget Fibre in Your Diet*, London: Martin Dunitz, 1979.

P. 178 *Australian researchers have:* Schumann, D. et al., "Low fermentable, oligodimonosacharides and polyol diet in the treatment of irritable bowel syndrome: A systematic review and meta-analysis," *Nutrition* 45 (Jan. 2018): 24–31.

P. 180 *In a smaller study, pectin showed*: Turati, F. et al., "Fruit and vegetables and cancer risk: a review of southern European studies," *British Journal of Nutrition* 113 (Apr. 2015): 102–110.

P. 180 *The person who can cope*: Dewulff, E. M., "Insight into the prebiotic concept: lessons from an exploratory, double blind intervention study with inulin-type fructans in obese women," *Gut* 8 (Aug. 2013): 1112–1121.

P. 181 *40 volunteers*: Pourhassem, G. B., et al., "Effects of High Performance Inulin Supplementation on Glycemic Control and Antioxidant Status in Women with Type 2 Diabetes," *Diabetes & Metabolism Journal* 37 (Apr. 2013): 140–148.

P. 182 *A daily consumption of 1/2 to 1 ounce (15–30 g)*: Maki, K. C., et al., "Resistant starch from high-amylose maize increases insulin sensitivity in overweight and obese men," *Journal of Nutrition* 142, no. 4 (Apr. 2012): 717–723.

P. 185, 186 *The solution was presented in 1994*: Lier, D., and M. Müller, "Fermentation of fructans by epiphytic lactic acid bacteria," *Journal of Applied Bacteriology* 76, no. 4 (April 1994): 406–411.

P. 195 *One study showed DNA from disease-producing intestinal bacteria*: Wang, F. et al., "Gut bacterial translocation is associated with micro-inflammation in end-stage renal disease patients," *Nephrology* (Carlton) 17 (Nov. 2012): 733–738.

P. 195 *Leakage of bacterial toxins*: Pham, N. M. et al., "Removal of the protein-bound solutes indican and p-cresol sulfate by peritoneal dialysis," *Clinical Journal of the American Society of Nephrology* (CJASN) 3, no. 1 (Jan. 2008): 85–90.

P. 196 *Already in the probiotics' infancy*: Siemenhoff, M. L. et al., "Biomodulation of the toxic and nutritional effects of small bowel bacterial over-growth in end-stage kidney disease using freeze-dried *Lactobacillus acidophilus*," *Mineral and Electrolyte Metabolism* 22, no. 1–3 (1996): 92–96.

P. 196 *Later studies show that*: Meyers, B. K., et al., "p-Cresyl sulfate serum concentrations in haemodialysis patients are reduced by the prebiotic oligofructose-enriched inulin," *Nephrol Dial Transplant* 25, no. 1 (Jan. 2010): 219–224.

P. 196 *Even though there were evident limits*: Nakabayashi, I. et al., "Effects of synbiotic treatment on serum level of p-cresol in haemodialysis patients: a preliminary study," *Nephrol Dial Transplant* 26, no. 3 (Mar. 2011): 1094–1098.

p. 197 *Despite the aforementioned studies' restriction*: Rossi, M., et al., "Pre-, pro- and synbiotics: do they have a role in reducing uremic toxins? A systematic review and meta-analysis," *International Journal of Nephrology* (2012).

P. 197 *A study from 2015*: Wang, I. K., et al., "The effect of probiotics on serum levels of cytokine and endotoxin in peritoneal dialysis patients: a randomised, double-blind, placebo-controlled trial," *Beneficial Microbes* 6, no. 4 (Feb. 2015): 423–430.

P. 197 *The dialysis ability to eliminate these*: Davenport, A., "How can dialyzer designs improve solute clearances for hemodialysis patients?," *Hemodialysis International* 18, no. 1 (Oct. 2014): 43–47.

P. 197 *According to Sirich m. fl*: Sirich, T. L., "Dietary protein and fiber in end stage renal disease," *Seminars in Dialysis* 28, no. 1 (Jan.–Feb. 2015): 75-80; Sirich, T. L., et al., "Effect of increasing dietary fiber on plasma levels of colon-derived solutes in hemodialysis patients," *Clinical Journal of The American Society of Nephrology* (CJASN) 9, no. 5 (Sept. 2014): 1603-1610; "Protein-bound molecules: a large family of bad character," *Seminars in Nephrology* 34, no. 2 (March 2014): 106–117.

P. 198 *According to a study looking at approximately 20,000 individuals*: Millichap, J. G., and M. M. Yee, "The diet factor in attention-deficit/hyperactivity disorder," *Pediatrics* 129, no. 2 (Feb. 2012): 330–337.

P. 200 *A WHO report asserts*: World Health Organization, "Public health impact of chemicals: knowns and unknowns," 2016. who.int/ipcs/publications/chemicals-public-health-impact/en/.

P. 201 *In the medical literature*: Bengmark, S., "The breast implant scandal shows weaknesses in the European information communication," *Läkartidningen* 109, no. 9 (2012): 485.

P. 202 *Researchers from Berkeley, California*: University of California, Berkeley, "Pesticides in Organic Farming," ocf.berkehtmlley.edu/~lhom/organictext.

P. 203 *This is exactly what is discovered*: Stefka, A. T., "Commensal bacteria protect against food allergen sensitization," *Proceedings of the National Academy of Sciences of the United States of America* 111, no. 36 (Sept. 2014): 13145–13150.

P. 203 [not 204] *Unfortunately it is on the increase*: Cao, S., "The role of commensal bacteria in the regulation of sensitization to food allergens," *FEBS letters* 588, no. 22 (Nov. 2014): 4258–4266.

P. 204 *Among observed results*: Yu, J., et al., "The Effects of *Lactobacillus rhamnosus* on the Prevention of Asthma in a Murine Model," *Asthma and Immunology Research* 2, no. 3 (July 2010): 199–205.

P. 204 *We also know that allergic children*: Böttcher, M. F., et al., "Microflora associated characteristics in faeces from allergic and non-allergic infants," *Clinical & Experimental Allergy* 30, no. 11 (Nov. 2000): 1590–1596.

P. 205 *As a prophylactic such children were given*: Aa, L. B. Van der et al., "Synbiotics prevent asthma-like symptoms in infants with atopic dermatitis," *Allergy* 66, no. 2 (Feb. 2011): 170–177.

P. 206 *You who have read Guilia Enders international bestseller*: Enders, G., *Gut: the Inside Story of Our Body's Most Underrated Organ*, Stockholm: Bokförlaget Forum, 2014.

P. 207 *He treated with repeated enemas*: Eiseman, B., et al., "Fecal enema as an adjunct in the treatment of pseudomembranous enterocolitis," *Surgery* 44, no. 5 (Nov 1958): 854–859. The last decade has seen a renewal in the clinical testing of fecal transplants. The method is practiced in many clinics, and it is estimated that between one hundred and one thousand patients are treated with transplants yearly in Sweden. This is according to Karolinska Institutet (Research Hospital, Stockholm), where they have an active research established in the field. See also: Hedlund, F., "Hellre mångfald än enfald," *Medicinsk Vetenskap* (2017): 3, ki.se/forskning/hellremangfald-an-enfald.

P. 214 *It continues to increase at the same speed:* Ann-Sofie Blixt and Maria Mejerblad note in their graduate work "Overweight and obesity in pregnancy" that "overweight and obesity is becoming an increasingly common problem. During a ten-year period the number of women already obese at the start of pregnancy have doubled. In 2005, 25% of pregnant women were overweight when they registered at the maternity clinic, and 11% were obese (Socialstyrelsen 2005—The National Board of Health and Welfare). This is to be compared with the numbers from 1978, when the number of overweight was 9% and the number of obese just over 2% among the pregnant women when they registered at the maternity clinic." (Brynhildesen, Sydsjö, Norinder & Ekholm Selling, 2006)." Blixt, A-S and Maria Mejerblad, bachelor's thesis for midwives certification, Högskolan (Polytechnic Institute), Kalmar, 2008.

P. 214 *Women with high BMI*: Mattsson, L. Å., and L. Ladfors, "Excess weight and obesity—a risk factor in pregnancy and childbirth," *Läkartidningen*, 100, no. 48 (2003): 3959–3961.

P. 214 *Anything that disturbs the process*: Blaser, M., "Antibiotic overuse: stop killing off beneficial bacteria," *Nature* 476, no. 7361 (Aug. 2011): 393–394.

P. 215 *It was the British Professor of Pediatrics*: See: Barker, D. J., "Maternal nutrition, fetal nutrition, and disease in later life," *Nutrition* 13, no. 9 (Sept. 1997): 807–881; Barker, D. J., et al., "Intra-uterine programming of the adult cardiovascular system," *Current Opinion in Nephrology and Hypertension* 6, no. 1 (Jan. 1997): 106–110.

P. 215 *A recent Norwegian study also shows*: Stene, L. C., et al., "Birth weight and childhood onset type 1 diabetes: population-based cohort study," *British Medical Journal* 322, no. 7291 (Apr. 2001): 889–892; "Maternal and paternal age at delivery, birth order, and

risk of childhood onset type 1 diabetes: population-based cohort study," *British Medical Journal*, 323, no. 7309 (Aug. 2001): 369.
P. 216 *The Finnish researchers*: Pärtty, A., "A possible link between early probiotic intervention and the risk of neuropsychiatric disorders later in childhood: a randomized trial," *Pediatric Research* 77, no. 6 (June 2015): 823–828.

MORE INFORMATION

www.bengmark.com
www.facebook.com/stig.bengmark
www.supersynbiotics.se
www.synbiotics.se

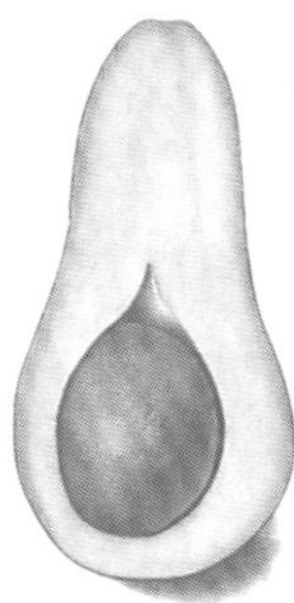

Originally published by Volante, Stockholm, Sweden, in 2018 as *Välj hälsa!*
Recipe photographs by Charlie Drevstam
Food styling by Sophie Berlin
English translation by Gun Penhoat

10 9 8 7 6 5 4 3 2 1

Library of Congress Cataloging-in-Publication Data is available on file.

Cover design by David Ter-Avanesyan
Cover images from Shutterstock.com

Print ISBN: 978-1-5107-6638-9
Ebook ISBN: 978-1-5107-6744-7

Printed in China